EXERCISE FOR MOOD AND ANXIETY

EXERCISE FOR MOOD AND ANXIETY

Proven Strategies for Overcoming Depression and Enhancing Well-Being

Michael W. Otto, Ph.D.

AND

Jasper A. J. Smits, Ph.D.

OXFORD

UNIVERSITY PRESS

OXFORD
UNIVERSITY PRESS

Oxford University Press, Inc., publishes works that further Oxford University's
objective of excellence in research, scholarship, and education.

Oxford   New York
Auckland   Cape Town   Dar es Salaam   Hong Kong   Karachi
Kuala Lumpur   Madrid   Melbourne   Mexico City   Nairobi
New Delhi   Shanghai   Taipei   Toronto

With offices in
Argentina   Austria   Brazil   Chile   Czech Republic   France   Greece
Guatemala   Hungary   Italy   Japan   Poland   Portugal   Singapore
South Korea   Switzerland   Thailand   Turkey   Ukraine   Vietnam

Published by Oxford University Press, Inc.
198 Madison Avenue, New York, New York 10016
www.oup.com

Oxford is a registered trademark of Oxford University Press

Library of Congress Cataloging-in-Publication Data

Otto, Michael W.
Exercise for mood and anxiety : proven strategies for overcoming depression
and enhancing well-being / Michael W. Otto, Jasper A.J. Smits.
p. cm.
Includes bibliographical references and index.
ISBN 978-0-19-979100-2
1. Mood (Psychology) 2. Anxiety. 3. Exercise therapy.
4. Exercise—Psychological aspects. I. Smits, Jasper A. J. II. Title.
BF521.O88296 2011
615.8'2—dc22   2011010216

9 8 7 6
Printed in the United States of America on acid-free paper

MWO: To Whitney, for her extraordinary love and warmth

JAJS: To Jill and Stella, for their love and support

ACKNOWLEDGMENTS

We owe gratitude to many people who have helped us complete this project. First among these are international teams of researchers who have documented the mood-enhancing effects of exercise in population-based studies, experimental investigations, clinical studies, meta-analytic comparisons, and review articles. We would also like to thank our collaborators on our own investigations in this area. In particular, our collaborators on research and review articles included Evi Behar, Tim Church, Lynette Craft, Lindsey deBoer, Daniel Galper, Dina Gordon, Tracy Greer, Pamela Handelsman, Bridget Hearon, Kristin Julian, Kate McHugh, Heather Murray, Mark Powers, Katherine Presnell, Georgia Stathopoulou, Candyce Tart, Madhukar Trivedi, Angie Utschig, and Michael Zvolensky. All of these individuals helped expand what is known about the benefits of exercise for mood and anxiety disorders. We would also like to thank Jaime Toussaint, Michelle Capozzoli, Michelle Davis, and Samantha Moshier for their help with drafts of this project. Finally, we want to thank Sarah Harrington, our editor at OUP, for her enthusiasm for this book and her expert help ushering it through the publication process.

CONTENTS

EXERCISE FOR MOOD AND ANXIETY

[1]

ABOUT THIS BOOK

There are many good reasons to reach for this book. If you have been plagued by moodiness, stress, anxiety, or depression, this is the book for you. If you are looking for a more action-based approach to mood management than that afforded by medications or psychotherapy, this is the book to read. If you have tried to exercise regularly and have failed, then this is your book. Why? Because this book is unique in focusing on how you can get yourself to exercise and how to make regular exercise a habit that lasts. This book offers a cutting-edge, research-based approach to integrating exercise into your lifestyle— all for the benefit of your mood.

We, the authors have published over 300 research articles on mood and anxiety disorders, and have over 30 years of clinical experience in helping people meet their personal goals. We understand the true nature of motivation. In this book, we provide readers with guidance on what underlies self-control efforts, and how to make the change process easier.

From population-based studies to clinical trials, powerful evidence suggests that exercise interventions can have substantial effects on mood, lifting everyday bad moods and feelings of stress, as well as offering treatment effects for diagnosed depression that rival antidepressant medications. These effects are powerful, and we open

Chapter 2 by presenting the converging evidence for mood benefits from regular exercise.

But how do you get yourself to exercise, especially when stressed, anxious, or depressed? Chapter 3 makes sense out of the common failures in exercise that are reflected in the broader failure of exercise in America over the past several decades. One reason for this failure is the substantial delay between effort and reward when one exercises for the benefit of health or body shape. Sustaining that effort, particularly when stressed, takes Herculean effort—as you probably already know. In contrast, when exercising for mood, stress is no longer a barrier to exercise; *it is the very reason to exercise.*

As part of helping readers adopt a new strategy for exercise and mood goals, Chapter 4 challenges the traditional perception of motivation as an inward trait that one must rely on for completing challenging tasks. Rather than looking inward, this chapter asks you to look outward at the actual determinates of motivation. We emphasize the active shifting of one's environment to reduce motivational effort, and we guide readers with rich examples of studies on self-control issues ranging from overeating to what is referred to as "effort fatigue." The result is that readers will be informed by the latest in social and clinical psychology research as it impacts motivation for change. You will finish this chapter understanding that reliance on internal feelings of motivation is a recipe for failure, and that alternatives are readily at hand.

Yet, how should you coach yourself around your exercise program? How should you think about your exercise during the day? What are the common thoughts that derail exercise? What should you think about *during* your exercise? How should you think about your exercise experience after you are done? Drawn from the success of the psychological treatment method known as cognitive therapy, Chapter 5 helps readers understand the power of thoughts for aiding goals and improving well-being. As a result, you will be better prepared to identify and intervene with thoughts that may hinder the adoption and enjoyment of a successful exercise program.

In Chapter 6, we focus on the challenges and solutions for exercise in the morning, the afternoon, or the evening. Attention to the timing of exercise and time management is complemented by a broader discussion of ways to make exercise a regular part of life. With this detailed accounting of common barriers and solutions for exercise challenges, you should feel ready to start planning an exercise routine. Chapter 7 provides the core features of our "exercise prescription." We chose to provide this prescription late in the book, so that our readers would have a full understanding of exercise pitfalls and solutions before initiating an exercise program.

Chapter 8 focuses crucial attention on the *feel* of exercise, and on those things that help individuals get the most out of an exercise session and the mood rewards it brings. The chapter addresses what you should think about during exercise, and how you should direct your attention between the pleasant and unpleasant aspects of physical exertion. We introduce a mindfulness approach to exercise, with the use of mindfulness to promote well-being during exercise, as well as the use of exercise to promote further mindfulness.

Chapter 9 then reviews some *do's* and *don'ts* of the post-exercise routine. How should you think about your exercise experiences afterward? How can you be vigilant to bad habits, such as compensatory eating and inactivity? This chapter reviews specific problem behaviors and presents a philosophy for change more generally. Readers are encouraged to adopt a practice of *echoing back* for themselves the enjoyable and achieving parts of their day. Although *echoing* is introduced as a skill for maintaining motivation for exercise, it is also encouraged as a broader strategy for enhancing well-being in life.

Chapter 10 focuses on the maintenance of an exercise habit. Boredom, social support, and seasonal changes get attention, along with practical information on motivational issues that emerge over time. We also discuss the role of family in exercise and the initiation of exercise interest in children. Chapter 11 then reviews what was learned as part of adopting an active exercise routine, and the use of an exercise routine to leverage additional health habits. We explain the concept of "health contagion" and discuss the importance of context in creating and maintaining change and well-being.

Throughout the book, we provide worksheets and learning aids for specific guidance. Also, case examples are presented, along with the authors' own experiences with the trials and tribulations of exercise motivation. In addition, to show that motivational challenges exist at every level of athletic performance, we provide commentaries from Olympic athletes on some of their own motivational challenges and solutions to developing a regular exercise habit. An appendix also offers additional information, web resources, and worksheets to aid your exercise and mood management goals.

Regardless of whether you are new to exercise or are returning to exercise after a period of inactivity, this book will provide you with guidance on how to approach exercise to benefit your mood. Our focus—and what makes our exercise prescription unique—is not on feeling good at some point in the future, *but in learning how to feel good now.* And just how powerful are these mood effects? The next chapter provides the answer.

[2]

EXERCISE WORKS
FOR YOUR MOOD

The mood benefits of exercise are supported by striking scientific evidence. Exercise can be as powerful as antidepressant medications in treating depression, and, more broadly, regular exercise is linked with decreased anxiety, stress, and hostility.

THE SCIENCE OF EXERCISE AND MOOD

Let's start with feeling good, and the evidence for the mood effects of exercise. To get benefits from this book, you don't have to know this information, but it does help to know just how powerful and reliable mood are the mood benefits from exercise. This knowledge can provide you with extra motivation for giving an exercise program a new try—not for your health, but for how good it can make you feel.

Part of the evidence for the mood benefits of exercise comes from large-scale studies of health conducted internationally. For example, a study of 55,000 adults in the United States and Canada found that people who exercised had fewer symptoms of anxiety and depression.[1] Other studies add to this list of mood benefits by indicating that exercise is also linked to less anger and cynical distrust, as well as to stronger feelings of social integration.[2] Yes, even better feelings of social integration—one of the benefits of regular physical activity is feeling more connected to others. And these benefits don't just include reducing symptoms of distress in people who have not been formally diagnosed with depression or anxiety. The benefits of exercise also include lower rates of psychiatric disorders; there is less major depression, as well as fewer anxiety disorders in those who exercise regularly.[3]

The idea that exercise can protect people against developing these mood and anxiety disorders has been supported by studies evaluating people over the course of many years.[4] For example, one such study examined over 10,000 Harvard University alumni over the course of over 20 years and found that rates of depression over time were linked to the amount of physical activity that these alumni reported.[5] Likewise, in a study of adolescents, 16% of those who were not physically active developed an anxiety disorder over a 4-year period, compared to half that rate among those who exercised regularly.[6]

Perhaps more important are those studies that have looked at how depressed mood improves once people start exercising. A recent study summarized 70 studies on this topic and showed that adults who experience sad or depressed moods, but not at levels that meet criteria for a psychiatric disorder, reliably report meaningful improvements in their mood as they start exercising.[7] Thus, exercise helps restore a normal mood!

A Note About "Normal" Low Mood Versus Psychiatric Disorder

So, what is the difference between feeling anxious or sad and blue, and a full-fledged psychiatric disorder? Disorders are defined by a group of symptoms that occur together, and that are severe enough and last long enough to get in the way of functioning. For example, major depression is defined by a sad mood and/or the loss of interest in most things, accompanied by a set of other symptoms such as feelings of guilt, low energy, concentration problems, disrupted appetite, agitation or immobility, sleep disruptions, and sometimes suicidal thoughts. These symptoms need to be present nearly every day for at least 2 weeks to meet criteria for a diagnosis of major depression. It feels really bad, and it is much more than chronic sadness: Depression is a self-perpetuating disorder that tends to recur. The latest estimates are that about 17% of adults experience a major depressive episode in their lifetimes[8] and that about half who have it experience recurrent episodes over time.[8] And, when it comes to those who exercise, rates of major depression decrease from 1 out of every 6 adults to only 1 out of every 12.[3] Not a bad effect!

There are lots of different anxiety disorders, but they have in common feelings of worry, avoidance, and *anxious arousal* (feeling keyed up, on edge, tense, and distracted). These various anxiety disorders are differentiated by both the focus of anxiety and what is done to try to avoid anxiety. For example, panic disorder is defined by recurrent panic attacks—sudden feelings of overwhelming anxiety that come out of the blue and are characterized by a rush of physical symptoms such as breathlessness, dizziness, pounding heart, and numbness and tingling sensations. The focus of the anxiety in panic disorder is on these symptoms, with fears of losing control, dying, or becoming embarrassed due to the symptoms. People with panic disorder try to avoid situations in which escape or coping would be difficult, should a panic attack occur. In contrast, in social anxiety disorder, the core fear is of negative evaluation from others. This fear leads to marked difficulty in social interactions, particularly with authority figures. Other anxiety disorders are defined more by what is done in response to anxious concerns, such as the repetitive compulsions that define obsessive compulsive disorder, or the daily worry that defines generalized anxiety disorder.

As is the case with major depressive disorder, anxiety disorders are common, affecting more than 1 in 4 (28.8%) adults in their lifetimes,[9] and they tend to be especially long-lasting when people do not receive treatment.[10] Panic attacks and anxiety disorders are two to three times higher among physically inactive adults when compared to those who do engage in regular exercise.

EXERCISE AND STRESS

A number of possible accounts explain why exercise might reduce a person's vulnerability to depression and anxiety. First, it appears that exercise whips your body into better shape to handle stressors. Exercise in itself is a stressor—it requires effort, and it forces the body to adapt to the demands placed on it.[11] This sort of regular, planned stress may help your body be better at handling stress more generally. Your body is toughened up by exercise. In studies, this is measured by less physiological (heart rate, blood pressure) and psychological (mood and anxiety symptoms) reactions to a stressor in individuals who have exercised.

A nice example of this effect was provided by a study of firefighters. In this study, researchers asked a group of firefighters to take part in a simulated fire drill (the stressor task) while measuring their heart rates and blood pressure, as well as their levels of anxiety and negative mood. After this initial measurement, the researchers assigned half of the group to a 16-week exercise program (using a rowing machine) and asked the other half of the group to maintain their normal physical activity routine. At the end of the 16 weeks, all firefighters completed the stressor task a second time. Even though the two groups did not differ in terms of their physiological and emotional responses during the fire-drill task before the exercise intervention, they showed clear differences afterward. Those who went through the exercise program had lower heart rates and blood pressure, as well as lower anxiety and negative mood reactions.[12]

The role of exercise in helping people adapt to stress is particularly important given that stress plays a key role in both the development and the continuation of depression and anxiety disorders.[13] People suffering from depression are 2.5 times more likely to have experienced stressful life events, such as the loss of a loved one, marital separation, or medical illness; indeed, four out of five episodes of major depression are preceded by a stressful life event.[14] Exercise appears to help buffer these negative life events.

EXERCISE AND NEUROTRANSMITTERS

A second answer to the question of how exercise reduces vulnerability to anxiety and depression has to do with *neurotransmitters*. Neurotransmitters are chemicals responsible for communication between brain cells. One popular theory is that reduced levels of neurotransmitters, such as serotonin, play a role in causing or maintaining depressive and anxiety disorders.[15] Antidepressant medications, such as Paxil (paroxetine), are thought to work by helping rebalance neurotransmitter levels. In fact, drugs like Prozac (fluoxetine), Paxil, and Zoloft (sertraline) belong to a class of medications called *serotonin selective reuptake inhibitors* (SSRIs). These drugs work for both depression and anxiety disorders.[16] A number of studies have demonstrated that exercise may be the nondrug equivalent of antidepressant medications like these. That is, exercise increases serotonin production in a manner similar to the desired action of antidepressant medications.[17] For example, increased release of serotonin has been observed in animals both during[18] and following[19] treadmill running, and prolonged exercise results in increased serotonin metabolism.[20] Studies with marathon runners and untrained individuals undergoing exercise training have shown that exercise has similar effects in humans.[21]

The notion that exercise can help clinical depression as well as antidepressant medications can is supported by a study of 202 adults (153 women and 49 men) with a diagnosis of major depression.[22] Participants were randomly assigned to one of the following treatments: (1) supervised exercise in a group setting, (2) home-based exercise, (3) treatment with an antidepressant medication (an SSRI), or (4) a pill *placebo* (a sugar pill). Participants in the supervised aerobic exercise category attended three supervised group treadmill exercise sessions per week for 16 weeks. During each session, the participants warmed up for 10 minutes, then walked or jogged for 30 minutes (high-intensity exercise), after which they completed a 5-minute cool-down. Participants in a home-based exercise group exercised at home but were given the same exercise prescription as those in the supervised exercise intervention group. Participants in the antidepressant medication group received Zoloft with the dose adjusted depending on the person's response to the drug and its side effects. Participants in the placebo group received the same contact with a psychiatrist as did the participants who were taking Zoloft, but they received a sugar pill instead of the real drug. Importantly, the assignment of the pill groups was *blind*—neither the participant nor the psychiatrist knew whether the patient was receiving the medication or the sugar pill.

At the end of the 4-month intervention, analyses showed that depression levels for participants in the exercise and medication treatments tended to be lower than for participants in the placebo group. In addition, 45% of participants in the supervised exercise group and 40% of participants in the home-based exercise groups no longer met criteria for major depressive disorder after the intervention, suggesting that they had recovered. Importantly, these rates were comparable to that observed among participants in the medication group: 47%. As could be expected, after the study was over, the people in both exercise groups were more physically fit than were the people receiving just the medication or the placebo pill. These results show that the effects of exercise on depression are similar to that of antidepressant medication.

EXERCISE AND NEGATIVE THOUGHTS

A third explanation for the protective effects of exercise focuses on the value of activity, particularly in response to anxiety and depression. Central to anxiety disorders is the concept of avoidance. Individuals with panic disorder, for example, avoid the sensations they fear—rapid heart rate, dizziness, breathlessness. As we mentioned, they also avoid the situations where these sensations and panic have occurred before, or where escape may be difficult should a panic attack start—places such as movie theaters, buses, locations far from home, and so on. They may also avoid drinking coffee or watching a scary movie because of worries about the sensations these events produce. Likewise, in depression, people start to do less—they stay home or stay in bed instead of continuing to be engaged in social activities. One way to treat anxiety and depressive disorders is to treat the avoidance part of these disorders—returning people to functional activity and giving them a chance to learn that situations are safer and more rewarding than expected.[23] In the same way, learning to persist with exercise despite urges to avoid it (being active despite a certain contradictory feeling), may help undo the cycles that maintain both anxiety and depression.

Consider Steven, a 29-year-old who came to our clinic for the treatment of panic disorder. He had his first panic attack after he was fired from his job about 3 years earlier. Sitting in his living room watching TV, he suddenly felt his heart pounding, and he started to feel hot. This was followed by aches in his chest and dizziness. Fearing he was having a heart attack or a nervous breakdown, he quickly called 911. At the emergency room, he learned his heart was fine, that he was not having a nervous breakdown, but that he likely had experienced a panic attack. It wasn't long before he had another, and he soon had racked up several trips to the emergency room for help with his panic. He stopped drinking caffeinated and alcoholic beverages, fearing that they would make him feel odd and lead to panic. He started to avoid situations where he felt especially vulnerable to panic, including social gatherings. As his panic continued, Steven became more and more isolated.

When he came for treatment, Steven liked the idea of an exercise-based intervention; it fit in with his preference for attending to the mind–body connection and using holistic approaches instead of just using talking therapy or medications. At the same time, he was apprehensive because he was worried about exercise causing him to panic. During the first 3 weeks of treatment, Steven progressed from a stroll around the block a few times per week to a brisk walk every day for about 25 minutes. He attributed much of his progress to the observation that he felt like he was fine during these walks and that he felt really good afterward. During the fourth week, he started meeting one of his therapists at a gym to work out on a treadmill. It did not take long for Steven to complete 30-minute workouts that involved running at a heart rate approaching 145 beats per minute.

Along with his progress related to exercise, there were meaningful improvements in Steven's daily life. Days went by without panic attacks, and he became more involved socially.

At week eight of his treatment, Steven reported an experience that had resulted in a significant shift in his anxiety. He had taken a road trip with his friends the previous weekend. Being far away from home had been difficult; this was something he had avoided for a long time. He was not particularly excited about being crammed into a small car for 8 hours straight, but looked forward to spending time with his friends. About 3 hours into the drive, Steven noticed that his heart had started to pound. His initial thought was, "Uh-oh, this is bad." However, pretty quickly, he reminded himself of the workouts that he had completed in the previous weeks and realized that this feeling was no different from what he had experienced on the treadmill. He calmed down. In subsequent weeks, Steven made further improvements, and became completely panic free. He reported that he had gotten his life back.

EXERCISE AND TOLERANCE TO BOTHERSOME PHYSICAL SENSATIONS

The shift reported by Steven is something that has also been observed in a number of studies.[24] In these studies, researchers examined how exercise can result in changes in fears of anxiety sensations (called *anxiety sensitivity*, because individuals are sensitive to and fearful of bodily sensations of anxiety).[25] These fears are often fueled by beliefs about the negative consequences of bodily sensations. Common catastrophic thoughts are, "I'm going to have a heart attack," "I will lose control," "I will go crazy," and "I will embarrass myself." In these studies, researchers selected persons who were high on anxiety sensitivity and assigned half to a 2-week, moderate-intensity exercise intervention involving three 20-minute exercise sessions per week. The other half of the participants were assigned to either no activity or to a low-intensity exercise intervention. Moderate-intensity exercise was defined as brisk walking or running on a treadmill at defined heart rates. For example, a 40-year-old participant would have a heart rate of less than 108 beats per minute if assigned to the low-intensity condition versus a heart rate of 126 beats per minute if assigned to the moderate-intensity condition (we will talk more about heart rates in Chapter 7). When anxiety sensitivity was measured again after the intervention, it was clear that this difference in heart beats per minute during exercise made a meaningful difference in terms of reducing anxiety sensitivity. The best outcomes were observed in the group that worked harder on the treadmill. One interesting observation was that the degree to which anxiety sensitivity changed after only 2 weeks (or just six 20-minute sessions) of moderate-intensity exercise was comparable to what other researchers have seen with 3 months, or twelve 90-minute sessions, of psychotherapy! These findings are particularly exciting, given that anxiety sensitivity appears to help explain why people develop and continue to have problems with panic attacks and panic disorder, as well as with conditions like social anxiety disorder, post-traumatic stress disorder, generalized anxiety disorder, and major depression.[26]

EXERCISE VERSUS PSYCHOTHERAPY FOR DEPRESSION

Could exercise be as effective in relieving depression as psychotherapy, you ask? To get a more complete picture of the effects of programmed exercise on depression, we reviewed 11 studies that had enrolled adults with major depressive disorder and randomly assigned them to either an exercise intervention or a comparison condition.[27] The frequency of exercise in these studies varied from twice to four times a week, with a duration from 20 to 45 minutes. Comparison conditions included no treatment (waiting for future treatment) or relaxation, meditation or low-intensity exercise (stretching). The results showed that exercise resulted in big improvements in depression. And, when we compared this result to the results of studies that examined the effects of psychotherapy on depression, we found that exercise performs as well as psychotherapy in treating depression.

WHAT ABOUT THE DOSE
OF EXERCISE?

Studies have not yet made clear the dose of exercise (the frequency, duration, and intensity of exercise) that has the best antidepressant actions. Both aerobic (prolonged moderate exercise such as running, cycling, or rowing over time) and anaerobic (like weight lifting or short sprinting) exercise have been found to be effective for decreasing depression,[28] although moderate exercise is more effective than lower doses of exercise.[29] Accordingly, in Chapter 7, we have prescribed the dose of exercise that is recommended to the general public for good fitness and that is also found to be effective for depression as well. Also, as you will see in Chapter 7, the dose we recommend also stays below the level of exertion that makes exercise distressing to most people. In this way, we get the benefit of exercise while leaving behind one of the central complaints about exercise.

What Can You Expect When You Start Exercising Now?

With regular exercise, you can expect to be better protected against stress and to experience fewer problems with mood and anxiety. You can also expect exercise to be an effective treatment for major depression and anxiety.

Perhaps one of the most appealing features of exercise for improving your mood and well-being is that you can expect to see some immediate evidence of its effects. Although overcoming a condition such as major depressive disorder may require weeks of exercise training, each bout of exercise along the way comes with positive mood effects that can be experienced right away. No matter how bad people feel before and during exercise, the feelings after exercise have been reported as uniformly positive.[30] In fact, researchers have found that the immediate effects of exercise on mood and anxiety tend to be greater among persons who have high anxiety or negative mood levels in general.[31] As we will discuss in Chapter 3, this feature of exercise—its immediate mood-enhancing effects—offers a great deal of appeal as you are trying to develop an exercise habit.

Perspectives from Champions

Exercise is the best mood booster in the world, at least for me! I view it as my *me* time. For example, when I am feeling down, the workout tends to bring me back to a positive place. It also makes my body feel fantastic, which reduces all sorts of stress. All the way around, working out makes my life so much better.

Kate MacKenzie, 2004 Olympics – Rowing

You don't have to wait months for the effects of exercise, as you would in the case of weight-loss goals. As you exercise for mood, you will be constantly reminded of the benefit you are producing.

ARE YOU A GOOD FIT FOR AN EXERCISE PROGRAM?

As long as you have adequate physical health, there is no wrong time to consider exercising for mood benefits. Some people will choose exercise to manage extra stress (job or marital changes, family illnesses), as well as more prolonged stress ("All I seem to have in my life are constant problems that need solving"). It is important to remember that both positive and negative situations can cause stress. Divorce is a negative life event when compared to, say, a wedding— but, as many people know, the impending life changes and huge planning demands can make a lovely wedding a major stressor as well. For all of these stressors, having a backdrop of regular exercise can change the tone of your days and help make stressors feel more manageable. People report that negative emotions surrounding their problems decrease during and after exercise, that the "stress just seems to fade."

Other people pursue exercise for mood in part because they feel bad about their shape and body, complaining that they often don't feel comfortable in their own skin. Refocusing on the mood benefits of exercise, instead of the shape benefits, can offer a powerful new strategy that, as outlined in the next chapter, helps prevent some of the common reasons for exercise failure. For these individuals, exercise offers a way to feel physical and to get a mood and self-esteem boost.

For those with symptoms at a clinical level, exercise can help reduce anxiety and depression no matter how long you have been experiencing problems with your mood. For some, exercise is an early choice for mood management; for others, exercise comes as a next step in a long line of treatment options that have been tried. Here are some examples.

Todd is a married man who has long been bothered by low mood. He states, "Good things happen to me, but it just seems like I am always low. It's like being just under the surface of water. I can see everyone else above water, up in the sun. But for me, I don't get there very often. I am tired of holding my breath. I want to get up and breathe like everyone else." Diagnostically, Todd has what is called *dysthymia*—a chronic, low-level mood disturbance, accompanied by symptoms such as sleep disturbance, low energy, poor appetite, poor concentration, and feelings of hopelessness. Dysthymia is less severe than depression, but it still takes a toll on well-being and the quality of life, including the quality of relationships. Todd states that his wife is growing colder and more distant. He says, "I think she is just tired of me being in a bad mood; she says she has more fun with her friends." Todd also complains of feeling sluggish at work as well as at home. He says he used to be in good shape, but now holds lots of weight in his belly. He would love to get back to a more youthful feeling of being invigorated. He has been to his doctor and has been cleared medically for exercise. He is worried that his feelings of sluggishness might get in the way, but he is willing to give exercise a shot.

Joan has been in and out of therapy for years. She says, "therapy seems to help for a while, but then some of my old patterns come back, and I seem to slip into depression." When depressed, she reports that it is as if her system totally shuts down—no appetite, no energy, and extreme fatigue. "My therapist encouraged me to think about using my body more, to complement what we are doing in our talk therapy. We are hoping that by using both mind and body, we can get better at controlling my depression."

Scott has tried antidepressants. He has been on several over the past few years, and has recently found one that appears to have some positive effects. Although noticing some improvements, he feels like he has a way to go. Also troublesome to him is the weight gain that he has experienced with medication therapy. Scott and his psychiatrist agreed that exercise may be a nice addition to his treatment regimen.

Sarah has never been to therapy, despite feeling depressed for more than a year. She says that she has been fighting feelings of shyness and shame for some time. She has been trying to get herself motivated to go to therapy, but her shyness gets the best of her. She says, "it is just easier to stay home, and hope my mood will get better." For Sarah, an exercise intervention could be the perfect fit because she could stay home but still be doing something to help her depression. She started running on a home treadmill. After running, she felt more activated, and more at peace with herself. As she exercised across weeks, she felt more fit: "I have been wanting to lose weight. I don't know if I have yet, but I feel fitter. I feel better about my body, and my mood really is different." Sarah was not trying to get all the way to "well" with her exercise, but she reports that she started feeling better about herself and was much less depressed. She felt better enough that she decided she did have the energy to seek therapy, and she set up her first appointment.

WHAT EXERCISE DOES NOT TREAT

Exercise offers some terrific mood benefits, and it will work even better if you use other resources available to you. But at every point, you must balance what your body needs and the role of exercise in managing your mood with other resources that can help you.

Exercise can be combined with either medication or talking therapy treatments. Indeed, with physical action, exercise can balance the focus of psychotherapy, which is more on talking, understanding, feeling, and planning. Likewise, exercise can be the active form of treatment for those who have started antidepressant or antianxiety medications. If, for any reason, you don't achieve the results you desire with this program, we recommend that you consult a qualified health professional (information on additional treatments for mood and anxiety disorders can be found in the Appendix). Likewise, exercise should not be substituted for other problem-solving efforts, such as learning how to better manage stressors in your life. This is especially true if you find that your symptoms are worsening, or if you start experiencing suicidal thoughts. Suicidal thoughts are a symptom of depression, and it is important that you treat such thoughts as a symptom *requiring immediate treatment*. Also, throughout this book, we stress the value of moderation and variation. As we point out in Chapter 10, overexercise can also be a problem that needs attention.

In sum, we want you to find the level of active engagement in exercise that best helps your mind and emotions stay in balance. To help you understand how an exercise program for mood is different from what you may have tried before, we start out this program of exercise by discussing why your exercise attempts may have failed in the past.

[3]

WHY EXERCISE PROGRAMS FAIL

We know that most exercise intentions fail most adults. You probably know this as well. Regardless of whether you are a former member of a gym, you once took Pilates, or you used to pitch for an intramural softball team way back when, chances are good that you know how easy it is to let exercise programs slip away.

Although most programs of exercise ask people to work out for some future fitness goal, our program is different. We simply want you to have an active lifestyle *now* because it can make you feel good *now*. This is a dramatic change from what people typically seek from exercise—future fitness, especially with regard to weight loss. Having to work now for a distant future goal makes it hard to stay with exercise—well, that and the busy lives we all lead. This chapter is devoted to making sense of past exercise failures as you begin to plan for exercise success in the now.

GOOD INTENTIONS VERSUS HEALTHY CHOICES

Health behaviors—things like smoking, sleep, and diet—share in common a powerful impact on health by influencing obesity, cardiovascular disease, and most notably longevity.[1] Unlike other risk factors like age, gender, or family history, health behaviors are *modifiable* (you can change them), and therefore they provide a clear target for preventing certain diseases, both on a public and personal scale.[2] We all know smoking is bad for us, that we should eat more salads and fewer cheeseburgers, and so on. But despite this knowledge, most people find it very difficult to change their habits, including the amount of physical exercise they get, over the long term, no matter how often they're told to get up and get moving.

To illustrate this, we have reprinted here a figure from the United States Centers for Disease Control and Prevention.[3] This figure shows that, despite the running craze, dancercise craze, yoga craze, and cardioboxing craze, the percentage of Americans who are sedentary has remained amazingly stable over the past decade. Notice what is being graphed here—this is the rate of American adults who have *no regular leisure time physical activity*. None! And the rate is stable in the range of one-quarter to one-third of adults.

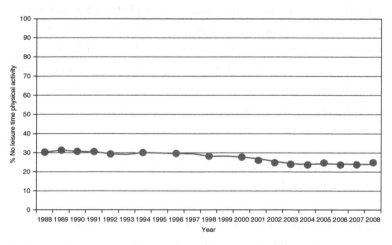

Figure 3.1. 20-year perspective on rates of adults with no leisure time physical activity.

Something that remains this stable for so long deserves our respect. There must be good reasons why so many people remain sedentary. In fact, we should expect these reasons to be firmly rooted in human nature. So, let's take a look at what we know about human nature when it comes to thinking about change, especially when thinking about making a change that is *good for you*. Allow us to introduce three key psychological processes: *focalism, fantasy effects,* and *delay discounting*. Here we go.

Focalism

Focalism refers to errors in planning that occur because a target task is not considered relative to other life demands and intrusions. Think back to getting your weekend homework done when in school. On Friday afternoon, it was easy to imagine doing your homework later in the weekend (let's say Sunday night) because you forgot all about the other demands and distractions of Sunday night. And, you probably ignored some of the problems with waiting until Sunday night to do your homework, like having access to the necessary reference materials for a report. It just seemed like a reasonable plan to wait. Then, wham! When Sunday night rolled around, it turned out that getting to the homework was as hard or harder than at any other time since Friday afternoon.

This focalism can have a powerful effect on all sorts of planning, especially when the planning is for events in the more distant future. By way of example, your authors routinely suffer from focalism around the academic assignments we take on. We are frequently asked to write chapters for other people's books. Writing these chapters is hard, and it takes time. We know this, and we often start out with a refusal, claiming that we are already behind on current work demands. But we are rarely successful in this refusal. We get fooled, again and again, by being told, "No worries, the chapter will not be due until this time next year!" When we imagine working on the chapter months from now, we see nothing but wide-open writing time. We tell ourselves it will be easy to do the chapter then. Surely, next year won't be as busy as this year! But it *is* as busy. The chapter has to be fit into an overfull schedule, just as we should have anticipated. We were too focal in our view of the future.

In the same way, future healthy changes look like they will be really easy. In contrast to making changes now, in the future it will be easy to quit smoking, exercise regularly, and take those yoga classes. Right? Future time always looks wide open; in reality, it is as busy and demanding as the present.

Fantasy Effects

Putting off a health behavior like exercise is also made easier by fantasies about the benefits. This is known as a *fantasy effect*. That is, fantasizing about the benefits of exercise (you know, things like, "I really will get in good shape. It will be easier to do things, I will look better in my clothes, I won't have the health problems my brother-in-law has, and my abs will look like Brad Pitt's in *Troy*") can reduce the motivation for exercise. It is as if the fantasy is satisfying enough in its own right, so our inclination to actually *do the work* is reduced. In contrast, accurate planning about the steps needed to reach good health is linked to following through with activities.

Here is an example. Researchers asked graduate students about their positive and negative thoughts on obtaining an appropriate job after graduation.[4] Likewise, the researchers asked a different set of college students to fantasize about interactions with a student they had a crush on, and asked yet another group to give their thoughts and expectations about grades in an ongoing course. The researchers also asked a group of patients awaiting surgery to give their thoughts and fantasies about the recovery process. Across all these diverse cases, the people with concrete expectations of success *and awareness of the steps needed to get there* had better outcomes. However, individuals with overpositive fantasies of success were *less* likely to get the outcomes they desired; they did not get a job, ask out the person they had a crush on, get a good grade, or recover well from surgery. Ugh, bad grades, dateless, no job, and limping—no way to be.

The lesson from this research is that the way in which people think about their desires may actually decrease the likelihood that they will take the steps needed to fulfill that outcome. So, to keep being motivated to get more exercise, don't get lost in picturing yourself with Brad Pitt's abs. Instead, keep your focus on what you want and the steps you'll need to take to get there.

Delay Discounting

Our third concept, *delay discounting*, refers to the way in which future rewards are made less meaningful by having to wait for them. In a classic demonstration of delay discounting, adults are offered different rewards—let's say cash—depending on when they choose to receive the reward. They can have a small amount of cash now, or a larger amount of cash in the future. All they need to do to get more cash is wait for it. But this is hard for people to do. For example, when given the choice between $40 now or $60 in several months, many people pick the $40 now. The value of the money in the future is discounted in our minds because of the wait. In contrast, the $40 now is real—it can be spent in the here and now. This is a tremendously reliable finding; books have been written about it.[5] You can also see this effect in action every April, when companies offer to buy your tax return from you for a fee (less money for you now, but no waiting for that check from the government).

Now, think of exercising for health. There is a promise of good health in the future—way in the future. Everyone would love a lower risk of heart disease, freedom from diabetes, and a slimmer waistline, but the effort is required *now*, and these rewards are in the future. Also, good health in the future is probabilistic; it may or may not really happen. You could quit smoking, exercise a lot, and then get hit by a car. By comparison, lighting the cigarette and sitting down to watch the game on television can happen now, without a doubt.

Let's put these concepts together. Due to focalism, it looks like tasks will be easier to do in the future. We can see ourselves performing a healthy new habit like exercise without all the busy clutter that is our usual life. Also, we can picture how easy it will be and how good we will look once we exercise, but we aren't so good at picturing the effort it takes to get there. Finally, relative to all the payoffs that happen tomorrow or the next day, the benefits of those in the future have less pull on us. We have a good fantasy now, but the reality of working toward that fantasy is hard, and that payoff is far away. It is much easier to just turn on the television: *Law and Order* now, plenty of time for exercise later. Focalism, fantasy effects, and delay discounting: Put together, they sap your motivation to act for the future outcomes that you really do care about.

WHY EXERCISING FOR MOOD IS DIFFERENT

Here is the really good news. Although exercising for shape or for health makes you wait a long time for benefits, exercise for mood does not. Exercising for a better mood *now* can make you feel better *now*! Although it may take you a while to climb out of depression with exercise (most studies of antidepressants, therapy, and exercise look at gains across 8 to 12 weeks of intervention), you are likely to start feeling some of the mood benefits right away. In fact, much of this book is organized around helping you notice and make the most out of the *immediate* mood benefits of exercise. If you can just get yourself started on an exercise session, you can feel very differently within a half hour. This is night-and-day different from other health behavior changes, which require you to wait for the benefit you're working toward. To drive this point home, let's consider another health behavior example—quitting smoking.

Quitting Tobacco: Best Intentions Up in Smoke

Just like rates of exercise, tobacco use rates have been frozen at around 20% of adults for over a decade now.[6] And, if you talk with smokers (and we do), you often hear a regular desire to quit. Smokers know that tobacco is killing them slowly, but they would prefer to think about quitting smoking next month, when the timing would be a little better. The effort of quitting is best saved until tomorrow, or the day after. . . .

Occasionally, though, something will happen to make it feel like this week should be the week to quit. Something moved the motivation to quit up on the hierarchy of importance. We recently had one such smoker come into one of our clinics. His name was Robert. He was 23 years old. He smoked one pack a day and had been doing so since age 14. He says his friends were smoking, and he just wanted to give it a try. Oops—now he's been smoking for almost a decade. Peer pressure helped him start, but it has not helped him quit.

Over the past 5 years, smoking had become increasingly more unpopular. This sentiment was reinforced by new city regulations prohibiting smoking in public places, including bars and restaurants. But Robert kept smoking. Then, one day, his uncle was diagnosed with lung cancer, and Robert felt like it was finally time to quit. He said he was ready: "It is a bad habit, and I want to live longer." The smoking cessation program he was joining was intense. It involved three weekly visits for 15 weeks, focusing on identifying triggers that made Robert want to smoke, developing appropriate coping strategies to deal with cravings, and learning healthy alternative behaviors. It was all free. Although it did ask Robert to do a lot of things that were new and not necessarily comfortable in the beginning, he said he was ready.

During the first 3 weeks, Robert showed tremendous commitment to the program, arriving early for sessions, having completed all home practice assignments. Likewise, during the sessions, he was involved and engaged, offering emotional support to other smokers in the program. Then came week 4. Robert did not show up. He called at the end of the week to let us know that he had decided to terminate the program. He told us he had lost his job, and that quitting smoking was no longer a priority at this time. He said that, right now, he felt healthy and that smoking didn't bother him that much.

Let's think this through. Robert wants the goal of future health. He knows that quitting smoking will help him have that future health. But quitting smoking takes effort *now*. It takes even more effort during a time of stress. And he is stressed, especially with the job loss. Stress and other negative emotions shorten our focus— we want relief now![7] Effort now for health benefits years from now—for Robert, this was not an equation for success.

But it could have been different.

If the *treatment itself* had helped decrease Robert's stress instead of adding to it, if he could have felt better with every session of effort, then he might have persisted toward his goal. His effort *now* would have reaped rewards *now*. And the stress would just make the mood rewards more salient.

Here's the thing: Unlike Robert's smoking cessation treatment, exercise can provide an *immediate mood lift*, especially when you feel bad beforehand.[8]

But hold on, you say, because you just remembered something. You recall how bad you felt the last time you exercised. It was punishing. It was no fun at all. Do we mean to tell you that there is a way to make exercise *itself* feel much better?

Yes, we do.

FEELING GOOD VERSUS FEELING BAD DURING EXERCISE

Research shows that experiences during exercise vary greatly from individual to individual, with some people reporting that they feel really bad, many reporting neutral feelings, and some reporting feeling really good. In contrast, feeling good appears to be the virtually universal emotion experienced *after* exercise.[9] One interpretation of these findings is that maybe you should try not to think about how you feel *during* exercise, and just focus on feeling good afterward. Not likely. Research indicates that feelings during exercise matter quite a bit when it comes to maintaining an exercise program.[10] Not surprisingly, people who feel bad during exercise find it more difficult to stick with their exercise program. The question then arises: Why do some people feel good, while others feel bad during exercise? There are several reasons.

The Intensity of the Workout

It should come as no surprise that feelings during exercise depend in part on the intensity of the workout. Positive or neutral feelings are more common during light- or moderate-intensity exercise than during strenuous exercise.[11] Indeed, much of the negative feeling during strenuous exercise appears to be driven by the physical symptoms of exertion.[12] With higher exercise intensity levels, the body's physiology changes, so that it can satisfy the increasing energy demands of exertion. That change in physiology comes along with all kinds of bodily sensations, most notably labored breathing that, in turn, often leads to a shift towards feeling bad about the experience. In short, maintaining an exercise routine is much more difficult when you exercise at an intensity that is (too) high.

How do people get to such high intensities? One reason is that they return to exercise with inaccurate expectations. For example, a memory of being able to run a certain distance at a certain pace in high school can lead a middle-aged person to set unrealistic goals. Running 3 miles in 25 minutes may have been a comfortable experience at age 22, when you were in great shape, but at age 40, after 18 years of relative inactivity, you are likely to experience this as especially strenuous (you know, about as much fun as being dragged behind a horse). Failing to appreciate the decline in fitness that comes along with age and inactivity may, in part, cause the negative feelings people experience during a return to exercise.

Focusing on the Negatives During Exercise

In addition, what we think about during exercise can have a profound impact on enjoyment and the likelihood of staying with an

> **Perspectives from Champions**
>
> You have to have the vision of what it is you are going to achieve by the hard work, but more importantly, you have to find a way to make the hard work fun ... every workout is a small competition within yourself.
>
> John "Big Jake" Carenza, 1972 Olympics – Soccer

exercise program. One handy way to take the fun out of exercise is to wonder how your body looks to others, or to worry that others are judging your body negatively. This bad habit is so prevalent that it has its own label: *social physique anxiety*.[13] Social physique anxiety rests on the assumption that others take notice of your body when you exercise and that they care enough to judge it negatively. The higher the anxiety, the more uncomfortable a workout when other people are around, particularly if a mirror is present.[14]

Discomfort with Physical Exertion

Also, people vary widely in how uncomfortable they are with the symptoms of exertion. To enjoy exercise, sweating and breathing hard needs to be no big deal. If it is a big deal, then feelings of fear and discomfort can arise and mar the workout experience. You read about this concern with symptoms in the last chapter, when we discussed panic disorder. That is, anxiety sensitivity (fears of sensations of emotional arousal) can intensify feelings of exertion into events to be feared.[15]

Fortunately, there are ways to decrease these fears. Our goal in later chapters will be to show you ways to get the most pleasure out of exercise. We will guide you on how to approach, how to think through, and how to more immediately enjoy your exercise experience. We will guide you toward a reasonable pace that gives you mood benefits but does not overwhelm you with feelings of exertion. We will help you to direct your attention to the pleasurable aspects of exercise, and to notice and drink in the mood changes that follow exercise as they happen. And, we will advise you on best enjoying your exercise benefits between exercise sessions. This experience of joy will help you stay involved with exercise over the long term.

With all these skills in place, all that is left to do is get you to try exercise. And, for that goal, we should discuss motivation, and how feelings of motivation work. That is the topic of the next chapter.

[4]

THE FOREST BEFORE THE TREES: THE TRUTH ABOUT MOTIVATION

When most people speak of motivation, they are referring to the experience of a positive feeling state when they imagine an event. "I am motivated to eat ice cream," means that, when I picture myself having an ice cream cone, I feel excited. "I am motivated to lose weight," means that when I picture the new slim me, I feel good. But a distinction needs to be made between *motivation for the outcome* as compared to *motivation for the effort needed to get there*. For example, there is a big difference between feeling motivated to become fit and feeling motivated to work out *now*. The first refers to the outcome, the second to the process of getting to the outcome.

When it comes to the issue of exercising for mood, we are confident that you have motivation for the outcome: You want a good mood—who doesn't? Our focus is on getting you to exercise, on the *process* of getting to the outcome you want (and not just the outcome itself). To prepare you for this process, this chapter provides a crash course of sorts on the nature of motivation, how it works, and just how malleable it is. With this information in hand, you will be especially ready for the strategies we offer in later chapters on how to successfully complete regular exercise.

BENEFITS, FRUSTRATIONS, HABITS, AND SELF-EFFORT

For anything that requires effort, it is important to understand the payoffs for that effort. Every day, for example, you devote tremendous effort to your work responsibilities. You wake up early (at least earlier than you would like), shower, dress, and then head out to face your day. If you have a good day at work, it all feels worthwhile. But, even if you don't have a good day, you know the payoff—your paycheck—is coming. You can continue to pay your bills and go out to dinner or a movie now and then.

Plus, you have habit on your side. You get up and go to work every weekday. You have the drill down. On days when you don't feel motivated, when the payoff does not seem worth it, you go in anyway. Habit often helps you accomplish your goals even when feelings of motivation falter.

But not always. Sometimes habit does not help, and neither does the payoff. Sometimes work is too frustrating and you find yourself face-to-face with the simple raw effort that you must apply to get yourself to work.

Benefits, habits, frustrations, and self-effort—all of these factors need to be taken into account when considering motivation and achieving your goals.

PUTTING IT TOGETHER: A BETTER MOOD NOW

Chapter 2 was devoted to telling you about the science supporting the mood payoffs of exercise. Exercise can help treat your depression, lower your stress, reduce your anxiety, ameliorate your anger, and enhance your well-being. Not bad, at least in theory. (And we recognize that it is *in theory* for you. We have told you it is true based on all the research evidence, but you have not yet *experienced* it to be true. Because you have not yet experienced it, it may not yet *feel true*.)

The focus of Chapter 3 was telling you about the challenges of exercise that occur if there is a weak link between exercise effort and the payoff experienced in the far future. We explained that there is a delayed link between exercise and improved physical health or body shape.

Now, to put these two concepts together. If you exercise to improve your mood *now*, you will not encounter the same delay in reward as if you were exercising for future fitness. If you exercise, you will feel different right away, giving you an especially tight linkage between the behavior and the mood goal. This will help fuel your motivation to work out. The catch is that you still have to make yourself exercise (and exercise at a reasonable pace and with a reasonable focus), so that you can enjoy these mood benefits.

You should now understand the theoretical linkage between the behavior of exercise and its mood goal. Once you actually try to exercise for mood, you should have a stronger, experiential linkage. That is, you will be more motivated to exercise *after* you experience the mood benefit for yourself.

Wait a minute. This sounds as though motivation often *follows* a behavior rather than *preceding* it. Is that right?

Exactly! The picture in your head of what exercise can do for you—the pull of exercise for you personally—will get stronger after you experience the payoff. Until then, it is all theoretical. "If I exercise, I *should* feel more motivated to exercise again because of the mood benefits I experience. But I won't know until I try it for the first time."

This presents us with a problem. What if you decide to wait until you feel really motivated before you start exercising? You may have to wait forever. Instead, to feel like exercising, you may have to learn strategies for manipulating your feelings of motivation. That's what we will teach you here.

LOOKING OUTWARD INSTEAD OF INWARD FOR MOTIVATION

Motivation is often spoken of as if it were some inward reservoir. Whether it is talking about one's level of motivation (as if the tank were either full or empty), waiting for motivation (as if it were an annoyingly late 8:15 train), or digging deep to find motivation (like drilling for a new oil well and hoping for a gusher), motivation is frequently discussed as a quantity. People may wish their motivation were higher, or greater, or they may lament their lack of motivation as if its absence were a personality flaw ("I guess I'm just not a motivated person"), but there is usually some sense that we should look inward for motivation.

In contrast, the exercise philosophy we advocate asks you to look outward for motivation. The trick is not in digging deep to find motivation, but in manipulating your environment to help you support certain motivations over others at any given moment. In fact, the best way of thinking about motivations is to think about a hierarchy of competing motivations.[1]

If anything, you are likely to be troubled by too many motivations. You have the motivation to sit, the motivation to watch a rerun of *Law and Order*, the motivation to have a juicy cheeseburger, the motivation to chat with a friend, and the motivation to live a long and healthy life. Think of yourself as constantly sorting and resorting your motivations. All of your pressures, wants, and needs are being resorted by daily and hourly reminders. Your motivation for food is enhanced by the wafting smell of steak tips coming from a local bistro. Your motivation to work late is enhanced by hearing about your cousin's promotion, and your motivation to do sit-ups is enhanced by the approach of beach season. Which one of these will win the competition for your focus and your behavior?

Influences on Motivation

Research shows that motivations are influenced by others—if a friend states a motivation ("I really want to get in better shape"), you may find similar motivations moving to the top of your list.[2] In fact, even seeing people walking in one's neighborhood appears to have a powerful enough motivating force that people exercise more when this happens.[3] Your motivations resort themselves, and your exercise motivations go to the top of the list.

Motivations are also affected by mood. If you become frustrated while pursuing a goal, motivation for obtaining that goal decreases, and other motivations begin to compete for your attention.[4] Even distraction can lead you astray. Research suggests that over two-thirds of women who have the intent to complete the regular breast self-examinations recommended by their physicians fail to do so because they simply forget.[5] Most of these women were probably very motivated to perform these exams while sitting in their doctors' offices, or upon learning of a friend's cancer diagnosis. But, somehow, their motivation decreases over time. This means that, for any intention you want to see happen, you need to provide yourself with reminders to keep the memory of your goals alive.

As such, part of success in staying motivated and following through with intentions has to do with reminders and cues that can help keep a specific motivation at the top of the pile. It is not about digging deep to find some hidden motivational reservoir; it is about working to have your environment support your intentions. This is what our exercise program is meant to help you do.

CONTEXT, CONTEXT, CONTEXT

In the book *Nudge*, the authors introduce readers to the concept of *choice architecture*, which is the design of the context in which people make decisions.[6] They make the point that there is no such thing as a neutral design. For example, if designing a building, the doors, windows, stairs, and bathrooms all have to go somewhere. Where you put them determines how people use the building, and it can also determine the building's ease of use, distractions and hardships experienced by people who work there, and general level of enjoyment of the building.

Likewise, how you arrange an environment makes a huge difference in the ease with which different behaviors emerge. Think of it as arranging the hierarchy of motivations a person has, using the environment to help move desired motivations to the top of the list, and trying to keep them there. And, how do you do that? Part of the answer is that you work to make sure that a motivation is not derailed by extra effort or frustrations or other competing motivations. Whenever possible, think about strengthening one motivation by using another to keep the desired behavior on track. You can leverage this concept in your effort to adopt a more active lifestyle. We will show you how.

Manipulating Environment to Support Behavior

Let's take the example of an important daily behavior (say, using the bathroom) and a problem that seems to occur across the lifespan for men: aiming accurately while using the urinal. Poor aim has quite a cost, at least for those who have to clean up. To help keep a public bathroom as pleasant as possible, and to reduce custodial costs, it pays to help men aim better. One option is to put up a big sign over each urinal: AIM WELL! Of course, to read the sign, men need to look at the wall above the urinal, and not at their urinal target. And the only motivation communicated by the sign is the management's desire to reduce a mess.

Compare this to the approach first adopted in Amsterdam airports and then later across the country: etch a picture of a fly into the urinal porcelain where you want men to aim. Manufacturers report a dramatic 85% decrease in spillage with this approach.[7] In fact, it appears to be such a good solution that fly etchings have spread over the Atlantic to public bathrooms across the United States.

Let's think about how this happened. Rather than relying on exhortations of good social behavior ("aim well"), the strategy took advantage of a natural urge to urinate on a target. In short, the fly etching co-opted a man's motivation to have fun while standing at the urinal. The manufacturers used the environment to help men want to aim well. We encourage you to apply similar strategies for exercise success.

Manipulating Environment to Support Exercise

Here's an example that relates directly to our subject: exercise. One of your authors got hooked on the Millennium trilogy of books by Stieg Larsson, starting with *The Girl with the Dragon Tattoo*. These books are exciting; they are hard to put down once you pick them up. In other words, I am highly motivated to read these books, but with a busy schedule it is hard to justify hours devoted to reading fiction. On the other hand, I am also motivated for the outcomes that exercise gives me, but my motivation for the process of working out is limited.

Can I leverage one motivation to get my other motivational needs met? Yes. All I have to do is let myself listen to the book in audio form when exercising, and only when exercising. The only self-control effort that needs to be applied is never listening to the book while not exercising. To help, I kept the audio book player with my running gear, and never put them anywhere else (to avoid temptation). As I wondered what would happen next in the book, I only had to wonder when I could have my next workout. Presto—I am motivated to run. In fact, it was hard to keep my runs short. I was repeatedly tempted to go just a little longer to see what happens in the next chapter. Again, the only effort I had to expend was listening to the audio books only during my running time; the rest of the motivation came naturally.

Let's review. I could say that *I should run.* I could try to drill deep for motivation, or wait, hoping for some natural running motivation to spring forth. And airport custodians could put up a sign saying that patrons *should* aim while at the urinal. Instead of relying on a *should,* I put my effort into creating an extra motivation to run. The audio book works like the etched fly on the porcelain. It combines motivations (one easy and one difficult) to make going on a run much more desirable. And, I get a double mood benefit—joy from the audio book during the run, and an enhanced mood after the run.

The number of additional motivators of this kind are many: getting a break from your day for fresh air, having sun on your face, leaving the office for a lunchtime exercise break, being alone to think, time for music, time for a friend, experiencing a nice day, or, when traveling, sightseeing in a different city. The key is thinking of your exercise time as an opportunity to satisfy another desire: What motivations can you combine to further support your own exercise goals?

SELF-CONTROL: THE EFFORT MUSCLE

And, what happens when space exists between motivation for the outcome and motivation for the process? Then it is time for effort, *self-control effort* to be exact. Sometimes only self-control effort can help you achieve your goal in the absence of motivation for the process. Self-control effort refers to the internal push you must apply to get yourself to do something. It is helpful to think of this effort as relying on a muscle—your effort muscle.

Just like other muscles, the effort muscle fatigues with use. If you work it early in the day, your effort muscle may be less available to you later in the day. The domain does not matter too much. This is a muscle that you use not only for exercise motivation, but also for other situations or activities that take effort. Imagine that you use the effort muscle to not eat all the French fries at lunch, and then use your effort muscle again to control your frustration and deal with a conflict at work. Your effort muscle will be fatigued by the time you try to make yourself pay bills instead of watch television in the evening.

The fatiguing of the effort muscle has been the subject of a fair amount of research. In a typical study, participants are stressed in some way, and then effort on a subsequent task is examined. The stress, or previous efforts, reduces self-control for the next task.[8]

AVOIDING EFFORT MUSCLE FATIGUE

Exercise is a way of training the effort muscle to get used to persisting even when tired (we talk much more about this in Chapter 8). However, when it comes to getting yourself to exercise, we want you to use your effort muscle sparingly. We want you to conserve your effort, and to use other strategies to help your motivation flow more naturally.

Divide and Conquer: The Value of Mini Efforts

For instance, one central strategy for conserving your effort muscle is to rely on a series of smaller pushes instead of one large push. Each of the smaller pushes is designed to enhance your exercise motivation and to put you in a context that better supports your exercise habit.

At each point, rather than digging deep for motivation, consider how to take a small step toward changing your environment, so that you get a more natural *pull* toward exercise from that environment. Consider the example of trying to motivate yourself to go running after work. You finally arrive home from work after a busy day, and you sit down on the couch to relax. The thought comes, "I should exercise." But from the position of the couch, it would take a Herculean amount of effort to rise and go running. The key is to avoid utilizing all that effort. Instead of focusing on getting yourself to exercise, we ask that you *focus only on the next step* that will make it more likely that you will exercise.

The first step is simply moving from the couch. For example, stand up, go into the other room, and change your clothes. You want to get out of your work clothes anyway—so change into your exercise clothes and then decide what to do next.

Once in the clothes, notice the feel of them. They represent a more athletic version of you. You can't help but remember working out when wearing these clothes. The running motivation is moving up in the hierarchy—help it along. The next step is to just get outside. You have been inside at work all day; wouldn't it be nice to be outside?

Hard way to get yourself to exercise:

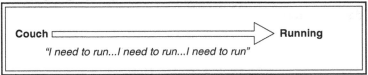

Easier way to get yourself to exercise

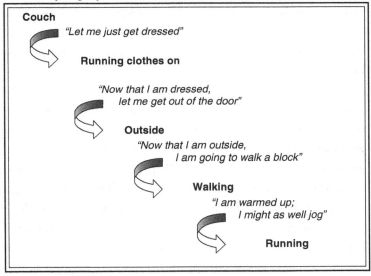

Figure 4.1. Figure reprinted with permission from Otto, M. W., & Smits, J. A. J. (2009). *Exercise for mood and anxiety disorders* (Workbook). New York: Oxford University Press.

Once outside, there is no need to break into a run—just focus on going for a walk. But, once you are walking, the decision to go running, and the motivation to make it happen, is much easier. You have saved your effort muscle from a lot of fatigue.

By using small actions to change your environment, you are chaining together small efforts into a larger gain. Effort is not applied directly to running, but to putting yourself into a better context in which to have your natural motivations take over, without an abundance of effort.

THINKING ABOUT EXERCISE

Helping exercise rise to the top of the motivation hierarchy—to win the motivation competition—also involves the way in which you think about exercise, including the way in which you remember past exercise sessions.

Let's say that, on the street, you see a couple jog past you. They seem to be having a nice time, talking with each other while they run in the sunshine. This cue for exercise can help resort your own goals, so that exercise moves closer to the top of the list: "I should go running later." But whether this happens, whether this momentary motivation is maintained, depends on what you next imagine. If you picture yourself running outside, enjoying the weather, it might happen. But, do you imagine that, or do you focus on the sweating ("I'll feel hot, be sweaty, and have to take a shower")? Do you get involved in comparisons ("I won't look as good as those people in my sweats")? Do you think about what else you may miss out on ("I was really looking forward to relaxing in front of the television")? Any of these pictures can help degrade your motivation to run.

Your motivation to run will also be influenced by how well you envision your last run (and the degree of well-being you felt during and after that run), as well as by your more general expectations of mood benefits from running. In later chapters, we program each of these aspects of motivational maintenance: how to coach yourself to keep motivation strong before you exercise (Chapter 6), how to focus your attention toward experiencing joy during exercise

(Chapter 8), and how to coach yourself after exercise to maximize your motivation for next time (Chapter 9).

REMEMBERING YOUR EXERCISE

People are not terribly accurate in their memories of their emotional experience.[9] First, they tend to overestimate the intensity of their positive and negative emotions. More extreme emotional experiences seem to be more memorable, compared to more neutral experiences. Second, emotional experiences are remembered with a so-called *negative bias*: not through a pair of rose-colored glasses, but through gray-shaded lenses that emphasize negative emotional experiences over positive experiences. Third, people tend to do better remembering the frequency of emotional experiences rather than their intensity; both are remembered inaccurately, but people tend to better recall the frequency ("I had three episodes of feeling bad") than the intensity ("It felt really, really bad").

In addition, there is some evidence that memories of an emotional event are biased by what happened at the end of the event.[10] For example, people may choose a task that involves a *longer* exposure to pain, as long as the pain is *less severe at the end* of the task. Really! It is as if the better ending colors the memory of the whole experience. The sense of relief that comes from a better finish helps provide a better memory of the whole episode ("That was not so bad").

A More Positive Finish Leads to a More Positive Memory of Exercise

Translating this into exercise and mood, how you finish your exercise is more important than how you start because the final few

Perspectives from Champions

I dislike working out until about 10 minutes after I get started. So, the hardest part is getting off my ass and getting going. To help with this, I plan a time when I will go, and then force myself to go then.

Olympic Gold Medalist – Men's Rowing

moments will disproportionately affect how you remember that exercise. In other words, if you can complete your exercise on a positive note, you will remember the experience more positively in the future, and this, in turn, will help motivate you to exercise again.[11]

This concept is really important, given that the toughest motivational challenge is often at the beginning of exercise. Once you get into the swing of things, exercise tends to get easier. Let's take running for example. The first minute or two of running, when your heart and lungs need to adapt to the exertion placed on them, can be a time of particular discomfort: pounding heart, breathlessness, and a sense of fatigue that may be qualitatively different from the rest of the run. Also, muscle tightness and soreness may be strongest at the start of the run, before your muscles have loosened up and begun to perform smoothly.

The take home message is: Don't end your exercise session when you feel overwhelmed with fatigue. If you are tired, it would be better (for your future motivation) to take a break (decrease your pace), so that you can finish your workout more strongly. In a distance exercise like running, walking, or biking, this may involve taking a break before you get to the end of your exercise session. For example, slow down and catch your breath before the last few minutes of a run, so that, if you want, you can finish with long plea-surable strides or a brief (very brief) sprint.

Again, why do this? Because giving yourself more pleasurable memories of your exercise achievement is both good for your mood and good for your motivation for future exercise—particularly, as research shows, if those pleasurable memories occur of the *end* of your exercise session. This is motivational management. By clearly attending to what works and setting it into your memory, that memory will provide you with additional motivation in the future. After you are fully enjoying your workouts, then you can play with more exertion if you want—but only if it makes you feel good.

USING HABIT

Earlier, we mentioned how sometimes habit can get you into work in the morning even if you don't really want to go. Habits are won-derful. They are automatic, easy, and, because of that, hard to break. We often think in terms of bad habits: Behaviors that have a natural pull and are so automatic that we have to be especially vigilant ("Uh oh, this is a high risk time") and work hard to resist them. But when the habits are useful behaviors, they can serve us very well for all the same reasons. Good habits, like bad habits, are automatic. We slip into them without thinking, without planning, and requiring no effort muscle. In other words, habits can keep us on track when motivation lags. Habits are like a greased track; all you need is a good nudge, and off you go.

So, how do you get your exercise to be more habitual? Regular practice, helped along by lots of reminders. One reminder is time of day—establishing a time of day when you will begin to feel like exercising (we help you with that process in Chapter 6). It may also include your set of workout clothes and your gym bag. These items come to mean, "work out." For this reason, pick a good set of workout clothes, something that gives you pleasure, and *never* wear them when you are not exercising (particularly when you are hanging around reading or watching television). We want the clothes to signal action. If you only wear these clothes when you work out, wearing them will make you feel like working out. And always keep these clothes in the same place, so that they are easy to find (so that you avoid the tendency to get derailed if you have to look under the bed for your cycling jacket).

Table 4.1. Exercise-supporting habits

- Exercise at the same time every day.

- If you use a calendar, write "exercise" in as an appointment.

- Have someone take an "after-exercise picture" of you and place this somewhere you will see it (e.g., your computer screen, refrigerator, by your bed).

- Keep a copy of your worksheet for monitoring your mood (see Chapter 6) where you will see it, so that you can be reminded of the immediate positive mood benefits of exercise.

- Keep other reminders of your exercise sessions (e.g., gym bag, exercise shoes, or exercise log) where you will see them.

- Wear exercise clothes that make you feel good.

- Never wear your exercise clothes when not exercising.

- Choose a place to store your exercise clothes and gear to make it easy to get out to exercise.

Let's give you an example of a similar use of cues around something that is really important to us: writing. Writing, and how often and how well you do it, is a lynch-pin for academic success. You can teach well, you can do killer research, but if you don't write it all up and get it out to the world, well, you will wither on the academic vine. Working up motivation to write is a lot like exercising for health. You know you need to do it, it clearly helps your future, but you have to work *now* for *future* benefits (and you know now why this is so problematic). On any given day, it is really tempting to avoid writing, to put it off until tomorrow.

So, how do you keep on track with writing? Let's take the example of B. F. Skinner, the Father of Behaviorism. By Skinner's own account, no matter what else he was doing, he would always try to write at the same time of day, and at the same desk if he could. He used both the desk and the time as a writing cue. He did not open mail at that desk, he did not read there; he only wrote at that desk, and only at the specified time. After enough repetitions, whenever he sat at the desk, particularly at the specified time of day, he felt like writing. It felt like the natural thing to do. Once he established the writing habit, he got an internal pull for writing from the time and desk cues. He reported that the pull was strong enough so that, when traveling across time zones, he would feel the pull of writing at the time when he practiced this behavior back home.[12]

In developing your exercise program, think about how to use habit—particularly exercising at a regular time—to make exercising easier, so that you feel drawn to do it. This is in contrast to using your effort muscle. Rather than having to rely on your own effort (push), let habit become a natural pull toward exercise. All you have to do then is put yourself in the right place at the right time, and you will feel your body take over with a pull of its own. You have nudged your exercise toboggan down the hill using habit.

Once you get this habit nice and ingrained, you can worry about diversification (diversifying, and avoiding boredom from too much repetition, is the focus of Chapter 10). Until then, the goal is to make exercise as automatic as possible, using your environment to pull you forward and using habit whenever you can, so that you don't have to use your self-control effort. Save that effort muscle for when you really need it.

USING YOUR TEAM

Other people can be a source of motivational support for your exercise program as well. It is clear that social support (having people you feel you can count on and talk to) is linked with better achievement of goals, including the ability to follow through with an exercise program.[13] In other words, having a supportive team matters!

Well before you start your exercise program, consider who should serve on your supportive team—people whom you would

---

Perspectives from Champions

Part of the joy of sports, of both workouts and competition, has been the team. Working out with other people feels entirely different from working out alone. There is a chemistry that happens that changes the feel of the workout. And the friendships that I have from rowing have a unique depth; we worked hard together, we laughed together, we won and lost together. That is a bond that stays.

Whitney Post, 1995 World Champion,
2000 Olympic Team – Rowing

---

like to tell about your intent to exercise for mood. A public acknowl-edgment of intentions helps people follow through with goals.[14] This is one reason why many self-help books ask you to write out your goals. This is also why we are going to ask you to discuss your goals with the people you care about and who care about you. Discussing your exercise intentions will enhance your motivation to follow through with your goals.

Your support team also serves a purpose in providing reminders for you to exercise, and as a forum in which to discuss

---

Box 4.1. SELECTING YOUR SUPPORT TEAM MEMBERS

Who are your support people, the people you feel you can count on and with whom you can discuss important topics?

_____

_____

_____

Who would be pleased that you are exercising, and would be fun to talk to about exercise?

_____

_____

_____

Who might join you in your new exercise habit, by exercising with you or being with you soon after exercise?

_____

_____

_____

your achievements. Sharing the joy from a good workout (by chatting about feelings during and after the run, as well as goals met for the exercise) provides the review and rehearsal of mood benefits that we discuss in Chapters 9 and 11. In the box below, record the names of people who are close to you who might serve you in this way. Think carefully about who to include, as not everyone is interested in seeing their friends exercise. Pick those people who can be truly supportive or who will want to join you in an exercise for mood program.

BE READY FOR LOW MOTIVATION CONTEXTS

In managing your motivation, it pays to know where your most difficult challenges will lie. These are situations that pull for anything but exercise. Just as those trying to quit smoking should steer clear of the smoker's huddle outside the building at work, you need to know what potentially exercise-killing situations or scenarios you must avoid. Perhaps one of the most high-risk situations, at least for evening exercise, is the couch in front of the television. There, exercise intentions can evaporate like a puddle in the Mojave Desert. If you intend to exercise, it is best not to sit down there. On exercise evenings, some people have a no-television rule until after their workout is completed; others avoid the living or family room altogether until after their workout; and some people drive straight to the gym, so that they cannot be tempted by the couch and television in the first place.

But this may not be *your* stuck situation. Take a moment to consider where your low-motivation zones are and what you might

---

Box 4.2. EXERCISE STICKING POINTS

Low motivational zones	Strategies for avoiding them
The living room couch	*Go straight to the gym after work instead of stopping at home first*

do about them. Think of ways to coach yourself out of them or how to avoid even trying to exercise at these specific low-motivation times.

Motivational Checks and Balances

In thinking about how to manage these low-motivation zones, remember that the goal is to manipulate your environment so that your goals are more naturally supported. Also, remember that the process of getting yourself to exercise can be complex. Exercising with a friend helps motivation (to skip a workout, you have to blow off a friend), but it takes the extra effort of arranging the shared workout in the first place.

As you may have guessed, much of the art of motivation is figuring out when and where to apply effort. Some workouts will be well-planned, so that the exercise motivations are kept firmly on track (a fun workout with a friend, with a clear expectation of starting at 6:30). Other workouts will not take this preliminary effort—you can just step out the door and be active. But, once out the door, you may need to do more to make the exercise interesting.

Your selection of exercise (running, biking, swimming, dance class, aerobic classes, ice skating, circuit training, and so on) is also important. We provide options for you to consider in Chapter 7; here, we just want you to be aware of the motivational issues, the *cost–benefit ratio* that best works for you. It is a good idea to balance ease of getting to the workout with considerations of the optimal joy

---

Box 4.3. AUTHOR PERSPECTIVE: CHOOSING YOUR
EXERCISE AND EFFORT

I run several days a week, but I don't like running. I like rock climbing. I really like indoor rock climbing, complete with padded floors, air conditioning, and music. Rock climbing is interesting, hard, and fun. It makes you concentrate. It gives you great abs. It gives you phenomenal grip strength. It does amazing things to your shoulder and back muscles. It gives you 2-hour workouts that feel like 10 minutes. It is much, much more fun than running. But it takes a special gym, a buddy to belay you, schedule coordination with that buddy, a commute to the gym, and specialized equipment. Running takes, well, shoes.

This is why I run several days a week. Running is easy. I can run to work, I can run in the morning before work, I can run in the evening, and I can run almost any time the temperature is not over 90 degrees (if you think I don't like running, you ought to see me running in the heat). Even though I don't like running, I like how running makes me feel—good. I like the time I have during running, listening to my music, being outdoors, and feeling the weather. I like the way running refreshes my thinking and relieves my stress. I like running in winter in snow, passing the cars that are creeping along and stuck in traffic. I like running when I travel, using it to visit a city up close and personal, on the streets. I like running in spring, looking at the blooms and feeling the return of warmer air. Okay, I may not like running per se, but I like what running brings me. I use running often as an example in these pages, in part because running itself can be boring. There are lots of ways to solve boring, and we believe that if we can help you like running, we can help you like anything.

So, as you read on, as we talk about running, please substitute in any other sport that you think is more fun and can provide you with sustained exertion. But if you don't love running, and this is the only exercise open to you on a given day, don't worry—we work hard in this book to teach you how to make regular walking or running interesting and rewarding.

the workout itself has to offer. (You will find that we frequently use running as an example of exercise and its challenges. We picked running because of these challenges—because it is a workout that, in our eyes, needs a lot of strategies to support it.)

PREPARING TO GET MOTIVATED

Motivation is a fluid process, with multiple motivations competing for your attention at any one time. Which motivation makes it to the top of the heap is determined by a rich combination of needs, internal states, external reminders, memories, and roadblocks. Each of these factors can be used to help keep a selected motivation near the top, so that you can realize your goals. For exercise, it is important to maximize the link between a workout and enjoying the associated mood benefits. The more you notice and review these benefits, the tighter the linkage between process and goal will be, and the easier it will be to get yourself to exercise the next time. In upcoming chapters, we get specific about this process, teaching you more about thinking and environmental strategies to make an exercise routine easier and more rewarding. To review, some of these strategies include making your exercise time a special time—time to listen to music, be with a friend, experience the outdoors, or simply to be alone to focus on your own thoughts and feelings. To get you to this time, we will have you rely on small pushes of self-effort. As outlined briefly in this chapter, we don't want you to try to get to exercise from the couch, but to use small steps in activity and changes in environment to help you more naturally get out the door in your workout clothes. How you talk to yourself during this process will make an important difference, and for that reason, we turn next to how you coach yourself in exercise and in life more generally.

STARTING WITH TARGETED ENDPOINTS

We started this chapter by discussing the difference between motivations for the endpoint (feeling good) and the process (exercising). The chapters that follow are all about helping you achieve the process (getting to and having good exercise sessions), so that you can get the endpoint outcome (feelings of well-being). But, before we get to the strategies, it will be helpful for you to get your personal motivations for exercise clear. Writing them out in black and white can help. In the space provided here, review and identify the symptoms you want to target with your exercise program.

Box 4.4. SYMPTOMS TO BE TARGETED BY EXERCISE

Please check off the mood symptoms you are targeting.

Symptoms of Depression:

_____ Sad or blue mood

_____ Loss of interest in things you care about

_____ Low energy and difficulties being motivated
to start or finish activities

_____ Feelings of agitation or lethargy

_____ Feelings of guilt about things done or not done

_____ Poor concentration

_____ Disrupted appetite or loss of interest in eating

_____ Feelings that nothing matters

_____ Difficulties sleeping or poor sleep quality
(or oversleeping)

(Continued)

Box 4.4. (*Continued*)

Symptoms of Anxiety:

_____ General anxiety

_____ Worry

_____ Feeling tense or on edge

_____ Feeling jumpy

_____ Startling easily

_____ Panic attacks

_____ Difficulties concentrating

_____ Problems with sleep

Other Symptoms You Want to Target:

_____ General feelings of stress

_____ Feeling angry or uptight

_____ Low vitality

_____ Feelings of frustration

_____ Write in:

_____ Write in:

_____ Write in:

[5]

DIRECTING YOUR THOUGHTS
FOR EXERCISE SUCCESS

All of us spend a lot of time in our heads. We are constantly thinking and evaluating, we compare what is happening in the world to what we think should happen, we review what did happen, and we anticipate what we expect to happen. It probably comes as no surprise that thoughts need not be true or accurate to influence our moods and motivation. Like most people, you probably have some bad thinking habits; you may have a habit of telling yourself things that *feel* true that are *not* true. This is especially likely if you are depressed or anxious: These conditions will cause you to view your world more negatively than is probably accurate. Intervening with these thoughts—learning to not take thoughts so seriously and learning to coach yourself more accurately—is effective for treating mood and anxiety problems. Learning to intervene with these thoughts can also be valuable in everyday life, helping to reduce stress and enhance mood. This can be especially valuable in helping you protect your mood and motivation for desired goals—like exercise.

This chapter is meant to help you learn how to detect and change inaccurate thinking patterns that will bring down your mood and interfere with your exercise efforts. We will show you how to watch out for loaded words and labels, how to "marvel" at negative thoughts (rather than buying into them), how to evaluate those thoughts, and how to coach yourself more kindly and effectively on your way to your personal and life goals.

THE POWER OF LABELS

A large part of all that time in our heads is spent labeling things. "That was good." "That was bad." "I did that well." "It was a disaster." All of these labels have an impact on how we feel. In fact, the labels we use help to define our reality.

Here is a non-exercise example of the power of labels. Researchers showed groups of people the same videotape of a car accident and asked them to give an estimate of the speed the cars were traveling when they struck each other.[1] But they asked this same question with one crucial difference between groups. Some participants were asked how fast the cars were going when they "hit" each other, some how fast the cars were going when they "collided" into each other, and so on—each using a different verb to describe the accident. Ratings of speed were different depending on which verb was used. Specifically, the average mile-per-hour (mph) estimates were 34.0 mph when the word "hit" was used and 39.3 mph when the word "collided" was used. The lowest average estimate was when the word "contacted" was used (31.8 mph) and highest when the word "smashed" was used (40.8 mph)—all for the exact same videotaped scene. This example shows that the use of a single word can influence the way a person assesses and feels about something. Labels matter. So, the next time you put a label on a performance or an experience, think about whether that label is fair. In most cases, it will not be, as labels tend to sum up only part of an experience, making the experience seem like it was one way or another, rather than a complex mix of experiences.

And, if you use a negative label ("My exercise was lousy"), then your feelings of motivation will suffer from the effects of this label.

Let us emphasize this point more clearly: Don't use loaded words as labels! Specifically, we want you to identify and stop using unfairly loaded words in your self-evaluations. Words like "disaster, horrible, worthless, and failure," are almost never true. Things may not be "spectacular, wonderful, and unbelievably good" either, so part of the answer is finding the middle ground. Good self-evaluation involves noticing the good along with the bad, guiding yourself more effectively and honestly. To be useful, self-evaluation needs to be accurate and directed at facilitating useful change (what can happen differently next time to make things better?).

SELF-COACHING

As you start your exercise program, do some work to clean up your thinking. We are suggesting this because of one central fact: Your thoughts do not need to be accurate to have a powerful impact on your mood and motivation. Think about the car speed study. People just like you made speed estimates that were almost 30% higher just because of one little word. This one word ("smashed") trumped the truth people were seeing on the screen. So, if you come out of a meeting (say, with a friend or with a work group) and think to yourself, "That meeting was a disaster," you will be biased toward storing and remembering feelings appropriate to that word "disaster." If you come out of the meeting and say, "Parts of that meeting did not go well," you will store and recall a very different emotional reaction. Likewise, if you exercise and run more slowly than you wanted, then say to yourself, "That run was horrible," you will be creating a dramatically different motivation for your next run than if you said,

"I was slow out there today, but I completed my 30 minutes." If labels can help or hurt your mood and motivation, why not use accurate labels that nevertheless put a more positive spin on the experience?

This is probably a good moment to mention Stuart Smalley. Stuart Smalley is a character brought to *Saturday Night Live* by Al Franken. In the Stuart Smalley skits, Franken delivers a signature line with sticky sweetness, "I am good enough, I am smart enough, and doggone it, people like me." This send-up of overpositive affirmations provides a good contrast for our goal for your thoughts. Just as we do not want overnegative thinking, we also do not want overpositive thinking. We want *accurate* thinking. More precisely, you need to develop an accurate and useful style for *self-coaching*—the way you talk to yourself in your head.

As you may have guessed, our internal dialog with ourselves plays a big part in how we perceive our exercise performance and success. You can imagine that, for a book on exercise, self-coaching is going to be important. How you talk to yourself is going to make a substantial difference for your motivation to exercise, as well as some of your feelings of pleasure after your exercise. More generally, how you talk to yourself is also going to make a big difference for your mood. This is especially important if you are reading this book not just to improve your sense of well-being but also to help relieve depression or anxiety. With these strong emotions, how you coach yourself really matters.

BIASED THINKING: THE INFLUENCE OF ANXIETY AND DEPRESSION

Depression and anxiety can bias our thinking and impact the way we label things, events, and experiences. In both disorders, people become more vigilant to negative events. That is, if you are depressed, you notice more negative things about the world.[2] If you are anxious, you are especially adept at noticing and reacting to threatening aspects of the world.[3] Also, once anxious and depressed, people tend to coach themselves in ways that maintain these disorders. It is as if the disorders take on a voice of their own. When down and depressed, people tend to become more negative and more willing to judge the world and themselves in a black-or-white fashion.[4] The world is seen more in terms of what "should" happen, with a sense of failure waiting if these "should" expectations are violated. Also, problem solving abilities decrease, and people lose some of their buffers against stress.[5] Instead of having a stressful day, people start having *distress filled* days. This is one of the costs of depression, and these patterns help maintain depression over time.

Similar patterns are evident for the anxiety disorders. Worries increase, as do expectations of catastrophic outcomes. Thinking patterns start being dominated by "what if" thoughts, where all kinds of threatening outcomes are both imagined and feel true. Two primary themes emerge in these thinking patterns: (1) overestimations of the likelihood of negative outcomes (confusing a remote *possibility* with a *probability* that something negative will happen), (2) and overestimations of the degree of catastrophe of these outcomes ("It will be a disaster; I couldn't cope"). Together, these two patterns enhance distress, and can make a person feel like danger is imminent.

Consider overestimates of the probability of a negative outcome like, say, a plane crash. For the phobic individual, an air flight feels life-threatening, even though the odds of crashing are tiny. Specifically, the odds of being killed on any single flight is on the order of 1 in 9.2 million.[6] It is possible, but it is very, very, very unlikely. Nonetheless, for the anxious person, this possibility feels likely.

Once a person becomes anxious, it is easier for negative thoughts to feel true. This is because emotions are like mood music for a movie. Mood music makes whatever is happening on the screen feel true. We get swept up in the story, and may only realize later that the story line was less than compelling. Likewise, our emotions make emotion-laden thoughts feel true. When anxious, it may feel unbearable to let the kids play in the front yard, with worries that they will dart out in the street. But when calm, you may recall that your kids know well to stay far from the street.

Our memory processes work along with this effect; emotions serve as memory cues. That is, emotions act as a bridge to other memories of when you have felt similarly. So, when you are down, you will naturally remember other times when you were down. This process makes it easier to have really negative thoughts ("Things have never worked out for me, and they never will"). Yuck. This is a classic thought that occurs to people during depression. When depressed, we really believe it. We believe it until we recover, and then we exclaim, "What the heck was I thinking back then?" In fact, correcting thinking patterns like this forms the bedrock of *cognitive therapy*, a powerful treatment for depression and anxiety disorders.[7] The techniques described in this book are meant to help you direct your thinking to better develop and maintain motivation and pleasure around your exercise.

The Tyranny of Dysfunctional Thinking Habits

Thinking patterns can become a matter of habit, just like anything else. Chances are that you have some powerful and old habits when it comes to your thinking patterns. Somehow, in life, many people learn to coach themselves in a way that is worse than the worst coach they ever had. It is almost like we resolve to be our own worst critics, so that no one else can surprise us with a criticism. Yet, who in their right mind would choose to spend all their time, day in and day out, with their worst critic? But this is what we do to ourselves, practicing these same nasty thoughts over and over again. Due to the repetition, these thoughts become automatic. We stop questioning these thoughts, which allows them to keep bouncing around our heads, worsening mood and torpedoing motivation for change. They can come to feel like an old friend—a really nasty old friend—but an old friend all the same. Old thoughts have more power than they should, and you likely have stopped questioning whether they are accurate.

Evaluate Thoughts Accurately: Marveling

Accordingly, a first step in changing thought patterns, especially old thought patterns, is learning to listen in and evaluate these thoughts. We want you to treat your thoughts as guesses about the world. Don't accept them as true until you get a chance to think them through. Old thoughts will immediately *feel* true because you are so used to having them (the old friend bit). For these thoughts especially, you may need a strategy for slowing down your thinking process. A strategy that helps many people is to practice *marveling*.

Marveling is a process of stepping back and having a sense of wonder at your thought: "Wow, I called that meeting a disaster; check out that word—*disaster*—that label sure could make me feel lousy and overwhelmed." That is marveling. Rather than accepting the label and emotion, you instead guide yourself to a sense of surprise and interest in the words you choose. This will help you obtain some perspective on the thought. Once you have this experience of examining your thought objectively, evaluate it. You may want to ask yourself one of these questions to help yourself evaluate the thought objectively:

- Is this really true, is [label/language] really the best way to describe what happened?
- If a friend told me about her own experience, is [label/language] really how I would describe what occurred?
- What is a more accurate description that better captures the richness of what just happened?

As you do this over time, you will come to learn some of the habitual ways you talk to yourself. Do you call yourself a "wimp"? Are you more inclined to label the things you do as failures, or no good? Do you keep yourself poised in an anxiety state by focusing on what could have happened ("If not for X, it could have been a disaster")? Once you notice some of these patterns, marvel at them: "There I go again." Then, firmly but kindly, continue with your effort to coach yourself more usefully.

To give you a sense of the sort of change we are aiming for, it is sometimes helpful to tell a story—to get yourself focused on someone else, and to decide objectively what sort of coaching may be most effective for you. So, here is a coaching story that has been part of a number of treatments for mood and anxiety disorders.[8] It provides a nice metaphor for how you can think about the way you talk to yourself.

A Tale of Two Coaches

This is a story about Little League baseball. It starts with Johnny, who plays in the outfield. His job is to catch fly balls and return them to the infield players. On the day of our story, Johnny is in the outfield and "crack!"—one of the players on the other team hits a fly ball. The ball is coming to Johnny. Johnny raises his glove. The ball is coming to him, coming to him . . . and it goes over his head. Johnny misses the ball, and the other team scores a run.

Now, a coach can respond to this situation in a number of ways. Let's look at Coach A first. Coach A is the type who comes out on the field and shouts: "I can't believe you missed that ball! Anyone could have caught it! My dog could have caught it! You screw up like that again and you'll be sitting on the bench! That was lousy!" Coach A then storms off the field.

At this point, Johnny is standing in the outfield and, if he is at all similar to us, he is tense, tight, trying not to cry, and praying that another ball is not hit to him. If a ball does come to him, Johnny will probably miss it. After all, he is tense and nervous and may see four balls coming at him because of the tears in his eyes. If we are Johnny's parents, we may see more profound changes after the game. Johnny, who typically places his baseball glove on the mantel, now throws it under his bed. And, before the next game, he may complain that his stomach hurts, that perhaps he should not go to the game. This is the scenario with Coach A.

Now, let's go back to the original event and play it differently. Johnny has just missed the ball, and now Coach B comes out on the field. Coach B says: "Well, you missed that one. Here is what I want you to remember: High balls look like they are farther away than they really are. Also, it is much easier to run forward than to back up. Because of this, I want you to prepare for the ball by taking a few extra steps backward. As the ball gets closer, you can step into it if you need to. Also, try to catch it at chest level, so you can adjust your hand if you misjudge the ball. Let's see how you do next time." Coach B then leaves the field.

How does Johnny feel? Well, he is not happy. After all, he missed the ball. But there are a number of important differences from the way he felt with Coach A. He is not as tense or tight, and if a fly ball does come to him, he knows what to do differently to catch it. And because he does not have tears in his eyes, he may actually see the ball and catch it.

So, if we were the type of parents who want Johnny to make the Major Leagues, we would pick Coach B because he teaches Johnny how to be a more effective player. Johnny knows what to do differently, may catch more balls, and may excel in the game. But if we didn't care whether Johnny made the Major Leagues—because baseball is a game, and one is supposed to be able to enjoy a game— we would still pick Coach B. We would pick Coach B because we care whether Johnny enjoys the game. With Coach B, Johnny knows what to do differently. He is not tight, tense, and ready to cry; he may catch a few balls and he may enjoy the game. He may also continue to place his glove on the mantel.

Now, although we may all select Coach B for Johnny, we rarely choose the voice of Coach B for the way we talk to ourselves. Think about your last mistake. Did you say, "I can't believe I did that! I am so stupid! What a jerk!"? These are "Coach A" thoughts, and they have many of the same effects on us that Coach A has on Johnny. These thoughts make us feel tense and tight, may make us feel like crying, and rarely help us do better in the future. Remember, even if you were only concerned about productivity (making the Major Leagues), you would still pick Coach B. And if you were concerned with enjoying life, with guiding yourself effectively for both joy and productivity, you *certainly* would pick Coach B.

During the next week, "listen in" to your thoughts to see how you are coaching yourself. If you hear Coach A, remember this story and see if you can replace Coach A thoughts with Coach B thoughts.

SELF-COACHING AND DEPRESSION

If you are exercising for depression, we want you to be especially ready to replace Coach A thoughts with Coach B alternatives. In particular, when depressed, it will be harder for you to notice and appreciate the gains you are making with exercise. Negative, motivation-sapping thoughts also will be more common: "Why bother? Nothing is going to help this depression," "Who cares! I feel so bad already; exercise will just make me feel worse," "I just want to be in bed; I will run tomorrow." Because you are feeling depressed, these thoughts will feel true. Also, they are likely to be accompanied by a host of additional negative thoughts about yourself and your abilities ("I blew it;" "I am no good;" "It never works out for me;" "Look at me, I am . . .," etc.), others ("He does not care about me"; "They don't like me"; etc.), and the future ("It won't work out"). Given that many of these thoughts are being driven by the mood (meaning, your mood is making these thoughts seem more likely and making them feel true), we don't want you to get too involved arguing with them. Instead, marvel at them, perhaps even accept them as background mood chatter—and then exercise anyway. Engaging in activity and exercise at times of depression helps to protect you from falling into pits of inactivity and isolation. Useful activity in the face of depressed mood helps undo the cycle of worsening moods and decreasing engagement that maintains depression.

To stay engaged, some people like to react to thoughts like these as if they were rebellious children. You understand why your thoughts want to go wandering off in the wrong direction, but you do not need to follow them. Guide yourself to useful action despite the presence of these thoughts. Regarding exercise, you may want to coach these wayward children by saying something like:

> Yes, it is possible that exercise will not work for me. And I know that staying in bed or lying down or watching television *feels* like a good idea, but now is my scheduled exercise time. I want to feel better, and exercise offers me a chance to do that. Let me get myself out the door to see how different I can feel.

Chapters 6, 8, and 9, respectively, are devoted to helping you develop a useful coaching style for approaching exercise, guiding your attention toward the most pleasurable aspects of exercise, and giving yourself full credit for your exercise achievements.

GUILT AND SHAME

We want you to be very careful about using guilt or shame as a motivational coaching strategy. Yes, we know other people do it. We know that some good coaches in your life may have dipped into the guilt or shame pile to motivate you. But don't do this yourself. Remember, you have to live with yourself every day, and it is rare for an emotion like guilt to lead you in a good direction. That is, it is just as easy to get mad and avoidant around guilt as it is to try to do the right thing. This certainly goes for exercise. Sitting on the couch and thinking, "I should exercise now," over and over again is a terrific way of making yourself feel bad and unmotivated. Instead, step away from guilt and shame and tell yourself the truth. Try something like this:

> I usually feel good when I exercise, but it is really hard to get myself to do it sometimes. How can I get myself in a position where I don't have to push myself so hard to get going? Let me just get up and turn off the television; then I can figure out what I want to do next.

Alternatively you may say:

> I feel busy, overwhelmed, and somewhat blue. These feelings naturally make me want to do nothing. But if I do nothing, I am left alone with these feelings. Feeling overwhelmed and busy is the perfect feeling state for exercise; it is exactly when exercise can help me feel very different. It is time to move, not time to freeze up.

Look at these two coaching strategies: no guilt, no "shoulds," just honest coaching.

A Note About Procrastination

And while we are on honest coaching, let us say a thing or two about procrastination. Procrastination—putting something off for an hour, a day, a week—really feels good in the moment. We need to acknowledge this. Stress decreases, but only for a little while. Then stress and other bad feelings increase. In fact, studies of procrastination[9] reveal that, although procrastination offers some immediate good feeling, over time procrastination both increases stress and

> **Perspectives from Champions**
>
> I continue to be amazed at the effect of exercise on my mood. Even just a short amount can greatly increase my energy levels and general happiness. Now that I'm not competing, it can be hard to convince myself to go for a workout, but it's worth it every time.
>
> Olympic Rower – Silver Medalist

lowers the chances of success. Procrastination also increases feelings of dejection, and is linked to a greater likelihood of illness. In other words, it is bad for you. We don't want exercise to contribute to procrastination. If procrastinating is a habit of yours, it will be important to set up a clear schedule of exercise. Then be especially wary of self-talk like, "I will get to it later." Remind yourself of the value of action; we want you to do it now as an act of selfishness—to save yourself feelings of stress, dejection, and lower success over time. Schedule it and do it. Give up the "shoulds."

SELF-COACHING AND LAPSES

Establishing a new habit takes patience and being comfortable with disappointment. As you work toward becoming someone who can say "I am physically active," there may be weeks during which you do not meet your exercise goals. Missing a spin class, skipping the planned morning run, or deciding that the week you are on vacation means a vacation from exercise can sometimes cause feelings of doubt or shame as it relates to your exercise routine: "See, this program is not for me," or, "Why can't I follow through for once?"

Lapses, or temporary setbacks, are common. We write about them here because we want you to be prepared to deal with them. Be prepared for surprises, things not going exactly as planned, and feelings of guilt or demoralization that may follow. Be careful that you don't take these momentary lapses too seriously by throwing your hands up in the air and saying, "Forget it. I tried this, but clearly this isn't for me," and discontinuing your exercise routine.[10] Instead, lapses are just additional opportunities for getting back on your schedule, for working to manipulate your environment to better support your intentions. When feeling demoralized about exercise, remind yourself of its utility—remember, bad feelings are never the reason *not* to exercise; they are *the* reason to exercise.

ENHANCING PROBLEM SOLVING SKILLS

One of the benefits of exercise is that it can both clear your head and quiet your mind, while also enhancing your attention and memory.[11] As such, exercise is useful for slowing down repetitive thoughts and aiding true problem solving (see Chapter 8). Now, all you have to do is make sure you get to that problem solving time. For that, we recommend a focused time each week. This time is used as an antidote to worry. Instead of half thinking about problems all the time, we would like you to pick a room and a time (let's say Tuesday at 6:30 P.M. at your home desk) to actively consider problems and issues for 30 minutes to an hour.

Rather than jumping from topic to topic, focusing on what *may* happen (the catastrophic "what if" thinking we discussed earlier in this chapter), this problem solving time is meant for focusing on clarifying the concern behind the worry ("What bothers me about this?") and how you might cope ("How bad would this be, and what are my options for dealing with this?"). The key is to stay focused on a single worry until you come up with answers to these questions. And it is important to write out both the questions and answers. Writing slows down the thinking process and helps focus it. You can then review your thought process, examining whether additional problem solving is needed or whether the worry itself is off track.

First, Define the Problem

In your problem solving, we want you to proceed carefully and slowly with problem definition. Many people skip this stage and set to working on solving a problem without quite knowing what the problem is. This happens frequently in the problem solving groups in our clinical work. Here is the drill. In the group, one member will mention a problem that he is facing in his life. Then, suddenly, like a pitching machine that is set too fast, he is bombarded by solutions fired off by the other group members. Five or six solutions come in from all sides, and the person with the problem sits there bewildered, answering weakly, "Yes, no, maybe, uh . . . I am not sure." His lack of enthusiasm is reflective of a crucial stage that was missed. The group, in an attempt to be immediately helpful, failed to help the person with *clarifying what is really wrong* and establishing *what sort of solution* is desired. This is important: Let us repeat it. It takes a while to clarify what sort of solution is desired, in part because it takes a while to clarify what the problem really is.

Accordingly, one of the first steps of problem solving training is to slow down this process, taking time to ask what is most bothersome about this problem. This is best done with a clear head, without worries swirling around and around—meaning that a good exercise session is an ideal prelude to an active problem solving session. During your weekly hour devoted to problem solving, grab a pen and a pad, and write out the problems you face (if you want, take notes on worries during the week and save them up for this time). Then, ask yourself the following question at least three times: What bothers me about this? With each answering of this question, ask the question again, trying to get more clarity. Only when you get to your third answer should you devote effort to the generation of potential solutions.

To help you generate truly new solutions (we are all such creatures of habit!), try to generate as many ideas as possible. Write down ideas that feel good, as well as ideas that feel really bad. The key is to generate ideas without devoting any energy to analyzing whether these potential solutions are good or bad. This is done this way because the process of generating a solution is very different from the process of evaluating a solution. We don't want evaluation to get in the way of generating new ideas. Only when you have generated new ideas should you pause to evaluate what is good and bad about each option (rarely is an option all good or all bad—remember the AND). Then, and only then, should you review the options you have generated and select the one you want to pursue over the next week. If needed, use the following worksheet to aid this process.

SUMMING UP

A core feature of this chapter is the notion that thoughts don't need to be true to have powerful effects on mood and motivation. Because of this, it is important to treat thoughts as guesses about the world, rather than facts. We have offered lots of examples of bad thinking habits, including the use of inaccurate and emotionally laden labels that lead you to tell yourself things that *feel* true but *are not* true. We asked you to start the process of learning not to take thoughts so seriously and to coach yourself more accurately. More precisely, we introduced you to the process of listening in on your thoughts and: (1) watching for loaded words and phrases, (2) marveling at negative thoughts rather than buying into them, (3) evaluating these thoughts, and then (4) coaching yourself more accurately and effectively. The next chapter initiates the process of applying these principles to self-coaching strategies for exercise, starting with the process of planning exercise.

Table 5.1. Problem solving worksheet

What is the problem?

Why does this problem bother me (e.g., what are the specific features that bother me)?

Is this a realistic problem (e.g., what do I really think is going to happen, and what part of this problem do I think is just worry)?

How can I rewrite the problem clearly, so that it helps me think about a solution? Write a clear restatement of the problem:

Table 5.1. (Continued)

Now that I have the problem clearly in mind, what are potential solutions to this problem? To generate solutions, I want to think about as many solutions as possible (without thinking why they are good or bad, and without choosing an option at this point). What advice might a good friend give? If a friend had this problem, what advice would I give? Potential options:

_____

_____

_____

_____

_____

Now rate each potential option. For each option, rate the good and bad aspects of the proposed solution. Do not select an option until each is rated.

Good things about each solution	Bad things about each solution
1.	
2.	
3.	
4.	
5.	
6.	

(Continued)

Table 5.1. (Continued)

Given this evaluation, which solution seems best?

Do I want to apply this solution, or is more time or more information needed to solve this problem?

Reprinted with permission from Otto, M. W., Reilly-Harrington, N. A., Knauz, R. O., Henin, A., Kogan, J. N., & Sachs, G. S. (2008). *Living with bipolar disorder* (pp. 64–66). New York: Oxford University Press.

[6]

PLANNING YOUR
EXERCISE ROUTINE

The goal of this chapter is to help you take what you've learned from the previous chapters and think through some of the specific environment and self-coaching strategies that can make it easier for you to get yourself to an exercise session. In doing so, we assume that there will be times when exercise will demand a more effortful push from you because of how it collides with your schedule and your other priorities. By the same token, we assume that there will be other times when it will take less effort for you to change clothes and head off to the gym, dive into the pool, or hit the road. First, let's consider some of the common roadblocks and some of the advantages associated with different exercise patterns.

MAKING IT EASIER TO EXERCISE: TIMING

When is the easiest time during your day to get moving and exercise? The answer is: whenever you want it to be. Just pick a time, and your body will adapt to whatever you want to do. If you want to feel like exercising in the morning, exercise in the morning. If you want to feel like exercising in the evening, then train yourself to do so then. Your body will pick up the habit.[1] The idea is to develop a rewarding exercise regimen that improves your mood and well-being. Exercise at those times that make the most of your motivation. Let's review some of the issues surrounding morning, midday, and evening exercise; examine each and pick the one that best fits your lifestyle and self-coaching habits. Exercise is easiest if you schedule it around (1) natural breaks in your day, and (2) times when you need a break in your day for a mood boost.

Morning Exercise

Exercise can be a terrific way to start your day. If you do it right, you can roll out of bed and be halfway into your routine before fully waking up. And, once you are in your routine, few interruptions are likely: Early morning exercise is often the ultimate me-time. Also, it can be invaluable to have a clear-headed feeling from exercise at the start of the day. During exercise, you will have time to organize your day, using the slow, clear thoughts that often emerge during and after exercise. It provides busy individuals with a jump on feeling creative, clear, and able to focus on the big-picture tasks of the day. These advantages may be one reason why morning exercise is particularly popular among individuals over 50 years of age.[2]

Another specific benefit of morning exercise is that the post-exercise shower becomes the morning daily shower, and, depending on where you live, the morning weather may be more optimal (lower heat and less wind) if you are exercising outdoors. Finally, with a good exercise session, you start the day with a sense of accomplishment, and that accomplishment can serve as a buffer against some of the other frustrations and stressors during the day. Against the chaos of the day, you had a morning where your effort led to direct payoffs—you put out the effort, and you finished your workout.

However, morning exercise is not without its challenges. One core challenge is the difficulty of getting out of bed early enough to allow for a full workout. With most peoples' schedules constrained on the back end (with a ticking clock until it is time go to work or school), even small delays in getting out of bed can compromise the time needed for an adequate workout. Also, from the perspective of a warm, comfy bed, a workout is an especially tough proposition.

Given these hurdles, if you exercise in the morning, it is especially important to chain your goals together for exercise success. The first goal is simply to get out of bed on time. Use the pull of other motivations in this process. Instead of thinking, "I should work out," think, "It is time to get up and go to the bathroom." This uses an existing motivation (assuming you have to use the bathroom) to help you get to a more awake state of mind and focus on your exercise motivations. From the bathroom, the goal is simply to get dressed in workout clothes. The clothes themselves give you a strong cue that it is time to exercise (it feels just plain silly to put the clothes on and not exercise). Once the clothes are on, the goal is to grab a drink of water, or a bite to eat (if you choose), and then get yourself out the door for your workout.

To help keep your exercise motivation on track, make this process as easy as possible. Have your exercise clothes and shoes out, waiting for you, and have your workout already planned. Don't allow frustrations or delays to make it harder to resist the thought, "I could just crawl back in bed."

To help morning exercise happen easily, be prepared to resist any of a number of motivation-derailing thoughts. These include thoughts such as:

- It won't matter if I stay in bed now; I can work out tomorrow.
- It is so warm here in bed; I will just snuggle in for a few more minutes.

- It won't matter if I miss my workout just this one time.
- My mood will be even better if I just sleep in.
- I am too tired to exercise.
- I can always exercise later in the day.

It will be hard to resist some of these thoughts as they bounce around your nearly asleep mind. Our principle is to never let a sleepy mind trump decisions made by an awake mind.[3] You made the decision to exercise on the previous evening when you set your alarm. This was the *awake mind* decision. Stick with this decision, regardless of what your *asleep mind* is saying.

Coach yourself through these moments by saying:

- I chose to work out now for a reason; working out early makes me feel really good later.
- Keeping my workouts on schedule does matter to me. I know I will feel better once I have started; time to get up and into my workout clothes now.
- Of course I feel tired, after all, I have been in bed. Once I start my workout, I will be energizing myself for later in the day.
- I am working out for my mood; putting that workout off until later in the day does not serve me. I need to get going now to give myself a better mood for the day.

Also, make sure you are ready for the motivation-sapping thoughts. Know that you are going to hear one or more of them, and be ready to ignore them. This is a form of inoculation against being derailed by negative thoughts. Look through the list above, and say each sentence aloud to yourself. Picture yourself thinking them while in bed on one of your exercise mornings. Then, picture yourself resisting them. And how do you do that? Tell yourself the truth about these thoughts: "I knew I would be saying something like this—I really just need to get out of bed and into the bathroom. Once I am there, I can think more about the workout if I want." That is, start your movement toward exercise success, and let this movement help remind you of what your *awake* mind had already decided.

Midday Exercise

One wonderful aspect of traveling in Europe is encountering the different tempo of the day, driven in part by the closing of stores between lunch and 3 P.M. This early afternoon break changes the workday from a long marathon of activity into two distinct half-workdays. The post-lunch break provides a way to be refreshed and refocused for afternoon and evening work. We like to think a midday exercise break brings these same benefits.

Afternoon exercise makes use of *circadian rhythms* that, in general, make us more ready for our bodies to perform physically well in the late afternoon.[4] This natural benefit, though, can be undone by weather challenges (e.g., the hottest part of the day) depending on where you live.

A particular challenge for afternoon exercise is disengaging from ongoing activities. Of special concern is the tendency to want to get "one more thing done" before exercise time. If you decide on afternoon exercise, you may well "one more thing" your way out of a full workout. Thoughts characterizing a "one more thing" tendency include:

- It will be easier to keep going; I am in the groove now.
- I am too busy to take a break now.
- If I keep at work now, I can have a really good break later.

Be wary of these thoughts. It may be well worth keeping your nose to the grindstone, as long as you can guarantee a good workout later. But be careful if you are missing scheduled workouts and not making them up. To help yourself counteract these motivation-sapping thoughts, remind yourself that exercise can enhance your focus and problem-solving abilities while reducing your stress (see Chapter 5). Think of exercise as your perspective time; when you come back to your work, it may feel very different. Thought-wise, you may want to coach yourself as follows:

- I am taking a break so I can be more productive later.
- I don't exercise every day, and so I need to keep my times. I will push for 20 minutes more, then make sure I fit in my exercise time.
- I am more productive when I take time to manage my stress and mood.

We should comment further on the last point. There is good evidence that exercise helps your thinking processes. When aged individuals are tested, fitness scores are linked to both overall scores of cognitive functioning (how well the mind works generally), as well as to specific attention and executive functioning (planning, decision making) scores. A wealth of studies show that individuals who exercise have higher cognitive functioning scores, but there is also reliable evidence that those scores improve with *programmed* exercise.

The combined results of 29 studies that tracked the exercise habits and cognitive functions of over 2,000 people found that aerobic exercise improved attention, mental processing speed, and memory, even in people over 70 years of age.[5] It's pretty clear that a high level of cardiovascular fitness not only protects the heart, but protects against age-related cognitive decline (*senility*) as well. And, the earlier in life you start exercising, the better the effects on cognition as you age.[6]

Briefly said—running is good for your noggin. So, if you are stressed or you have to perform well at work, getting out to exercise in the middle of the day might be a terrific way to get your work done, and done well.

Evening Exercise

We think evening exercise is a wonderful way to end the day, including providing a shift between work and social or family hours. This is especially important if you have trouble leaving work at work—if you instead take home worries from the workday that invade your evening hours. If this is your pattern, try practicing *door-closing strategies* to help you better segment your day. Before leaving work, pause to write out your concerns from the day and an agenda for addressing these concerns *tomorrow*. This is the last hurrah for the workday—to clarify how you will re-attend to issues tomorrow. Devote 5 minutes to this process, taking this extra work time to help make your evening cleaner. With this list written and left on your desk or in your drawer, stand up and formally say goodbye to the day and close the office door (either actually or conceptually).

Your exercise session can then serve as your transition time between work and home. It is time for you to clear your head and get ready to become your social or family self. For this purpose, exercise is completed *before you get home*. This helps you avoid all the derailing events that await you at home, including the television and couch waiting to swallow up your motivation.

Consider whether you can make your exercise part of your commute (by running, biking, or rollerblading to and from work). Having exercise as part of your commute is amazingly efficient. Biking, rollerblading, or running is a terrific antidote to the time you spend in traffic. Since you are commuting anyway, exercise time spent during the commute does not take time away from the rest of your life. Commuting exercise also makes your workouts feel very functional—to be at work (or back home) on time, you have to keep up a certain pace. And, even though you might like to stop, you do still have to get to work (or home) somehow.

Commuting workouts do demand a shower near work and the ability to manage clothes (having a change of clothes stored in the office, and a place to hang-dry your workout clothes, especially if you need to change back into them for the commute home). These workouts may be easier to arrange in winter, when sweating may be reduced in the cold weather. Because exercise this way involves a change of clothes and a shower afterward, plan for how these disruptions can best fall into your daily routine. Remember, the goal for your exercise program is to maximize motivation not by force, but by finesse.

If commuting workouts are not feasible, consider ways to combine your motivations for evening workouts. If you have a favorite television show, rather than watching it from the couch, consider watching it from the treadmill or cycle at home or in the gym. You make time in your schedule for the show by making it count as exercise time. Finally, if there just isn't time before you get home and get integrated into family activities, then think about how exercise can happen with the family (see Chapter 10). Running while a child bikes or using a jogging stroller can help family time double as exercise time, while offering the benefits of exercise to those you love.

For all of these approaches, be wary of the derailing thoughts that come in the evening. These often surround being too tired or too busy for the workout:

- I have had a full day; I am too tired to work out.
- It is about to get dark. I can just put it off until morning.

- I have achieved enough today; I can let the workouts go for now.
- I was moving constantly at work; I don't need to work out tonight.

Fatigue from a busy workday, even if you do physical work, is no reason to skip leisure time exercise. Work-related physical activities often occur at a low heart rate, and these activities, even though they are taxing, are not linked to either physical or mental health benefits.[7] They don't help, and they can be used as an excuse to skip a workout.

Coach yourself around your fatigue with phrases like:

- I am tired, but I can still have a good workout that will leave me feeling refreshed mentally and in a better mood for tomorrow.
- This workout is my transition to having a really good evening.
- With this workout, I will feel reset for a better day tomorrow.

Then, get yourself to your workout.

Perspectives from Champions

A workout is hard to start especially after a long day, missed meal, or seated at a desk/vehicle. I schedule the workout each day on the previous day. I make sure I vary the workout (cross-train) and vary the time of day. This seems to keep my interest in the workout; after a while, the workout becomes a good habit, something that I do not want to miss.

Daniel K. Sayner 1980 Olympic Rowing
(USA boycott)

COMMON EXCUSES FOR SKIPPING EXERCISE

Why do we skip our workouts, even though we know how important they are? Here are some of the most common reasons people offer to themselves for not exercising, along with techniques you can use to stay motivated.

Too Stressed to Exercise

Problem solving is often hampered by focusing too intently on only one way of defining the problem or conceptualizing the solution. With true problem solving efforts stymied, it becomes easy for thinking to become *ruminative*—the same thoughts begin bouncing around inside your head, again and again. Unfortunately, while these thoughts bounce around and around, they often pick up emotions (anxiety, sadness, frustration) that can further hamper problem solving efforts and increase ruminative worry. What you need at

---

Perspectives from Champions

Use exercise as an escape. No one will be yapping in your ear, and you will be alone with your thoughts. Don't overdo the exercise. If you are a 12-minute miler, then don't try to run an 11:30 mile. That makes you miserable and sore. Just get started, even if that means a 30-minute walk. If nothing else, you will sleep better and wake up fresh. Whenever I am super-stressed and can't sleep, I always up the mileage. Works like a champ.

Olympic Gold Medalist – Rowing

---

these moments is an emotional and cognitive reset button. Push this button, and the worry and thinking process goes offline, shuts down temporarily, and then comes back online in a fresh way, so that any of a number of potential problem definitions or solution strategies can be embraced.

In the absence of a true reset button on your forehead, a session of exercise is not a bad alternative. As noted earlier, we know that exercise can enhance attention and memory,[8] but in the midst of a bout of worry and stress, it can also bring about an all-important change in context that allows new solutions to emerge. As individuals who write for a living, as part of both our day and evening jobs, we cannot tell you the countless times we've been frustrated by a paragraph, spending tremendous mental energy trying to make a point clear, only to be stymied by all efforts. Yet, if we are wise or lucky enough to take a brief exercise break, a better way of expressing ourselves may suddenly leap to mind. There is nothing specific about the exercise in the process, except that it can help us stop ruminating about the paragraph long enough for new ideas to emerge. Exercise is the reset button: It stops the old process and provides an open road for new ideas. Also, being away from the desk also helps; not only does exercise provide a new venue, it makes it impossible to write down anything until the idea fully gels. All of these elements work together—change in venue, change in internal state, reset button clarity, emotional recharge—to give you a new perspective for tackling the next task at hand.

Too Depressed to Exercise

When you are down, blue, or sad, it is sorely tempting to skip a workout. But, as you hear yourself say, "I don't feel like it," remember that this is the very time at which exercise is most likely to help. Choosing

Box 6.1. AUTHOR PERSPECTIVE: TOO STRESSED
TO EXERCISE

Exercise. Why bother? No really, why bother? It is hard, sweaty, and requires effort and planning. So, let me tell you a story. It all takes place between these sentences and the next section. OK, not these sentences. The sentences I had written here have now been erased. They were boring, horrible little sentences. I was bored writing them, and I was in a bad mood. I had lots of reasons to be in a bad mood. I had a pile of stressors, I was behind on multiple projects, and my academic team was positively dripping with issues. And, I had to write this section. I decided to take a break. I had no desire to run; it was winter, and it was cold out. But I had avoided exercise yesterday, and I did not want to face how hard it becomes when you avoid exercise two days in a row. So, I suited up. I am calling it "suiting up" so that it will sound cooler than it really was. Like I said, I did not want to run, and I needed something, even a little false cool. I pulled on my decidedly uncool running outfit. I also grabbed my iPod. I went out into the winter air.

I started. My legs were heavy, and my gait was awkward. I told myself that I hate running. I listened to my first song, trying to get comfortable in my disdain. It was cold, but the sun was warm on my face, the music was good, and I was comfortable in my hate of exercise. I ran on. Somewhere after the first mile, my gait loosened (the beauty of running frequently is that the first mile can be ignored—you wait awhile, and the bad part just goes away). And I became more aware of my music. It was "My Baby

Just Cares For Me" by Nina Simone. Do you know it? The piano work is absolutely joyful. I leaned into the music. I felt some sadness pass up from my chest to my eyes. I let it sit there. And the sadness sat there until the next song, by The Fray—piano work dropping into rich guitar chords. I leaned into that music as well. The sadness and stress shifted again. I began to feel hollow. Not hollow in an empty way, but hollow like I was now letting something move through and out of me. I would say it was *energy*, but I am not from California. I felt better. I picked up my pace and thought about people I had not called and what I had to do later in the day. I thought about writing this paragraph. I picked up my pace. I listened to "Leaving on a Jet Plane" (yes, really, but it was by Chantal Kreviazuk). I felt open and full. I picked up my pace, I listened to more music, I looked at the ice on the pond, I looked at the bare trees, and I finished the run. I walked the last few blocks home. I wrote these paragraphs. I feel light. I feel good. My list of problems sits a few more yards away from me and seems manageable; the list will get attention, item by item.

not to exercise because you are feeling down is like choosing not to take an aspirin because you have a headache. The aspirin is for times when you have a headache, and exercise is most effective when you are feeling down. When you feel blue, we want you to think selfishly. We want you to want to feel differently, to feel better. And, we want you to use that desire to feel better as motivation to exercise.

Get right out there to your workout. Know that sad moods blunt motivation and make frustrations feel that much more annoying. So, make your workout simple, without a lot of planning—only a devotion to making yourself feel better. And when you feel better, don't forget to notice. Remind yourself how you did not want to exercise, and notice just how differently you feel. There is a reason why you take aspirin for a headache—make sure you feel the reason why you exercise.

Consider the following example. James was a 59-year-old married man with a long history of depression and suicidal thoughts. He had tried a number of medications, but had never responded very well. He had heard about exercise treatment for depression on the news and contacted one of us for consultation; exercise to overcome depression seemed right to him. In the first few weeks of treatment, the focus was on suicidal thoughts and feelings of inertia. Much of the work involved helping him shift his thinking away from a style that supported depression (see Chapter 5) and to start a process of increasing pleasurable activities. Within the context of activity goals, exercise fit right in. James had not exercised in a while, so walking around the neighborhood seemed like a good first step. When? Initially, we decided the morning was best as this would help jump-start James' day. His response to exercise was good; it had the desired effect of helping him "feel more alive." But James frequently did not meet his own exercise goals. After 5 weeks, it became clear he needed a better way of establishing an exercise habit that matched his mood needs. Through monitoring of mood, James noticed that his mood always took a down-turn at 5:00 p.m.—after a 9-hour workday. It was clear to both of us that this was the time of day when he needed an intervention. Now, exercise could be used in direct response to his greatest mood challenge.

To help you monitor your mood in this way, you may want to use a series of simple numerical ratings (on a 0 to 100 scale) to keep track of changes in your mood, thoughts, and energy level as you exercise. Seeing the benefit that exercise gives you will give you motivation for your next workout and will help you resist thoughts about skipping a workout because you are in a bad mood or fatigued.

Too Bored to Exercise

If your next workout seems like it might be boring, well, think about what you could do to spice it up. Which music? What location?

Table 6.1. Log for tracking mood benefits

	Very Bad	Bad	Neutral	Good	Very Good
HOW I FELT *BEFORE* EXERCISE					
My mood was:	0	10 20 30	40 50 60	70 80 90	100
My thoughts were:	0	10 20 30	40 50 60	70 80 90	100
My energy level was:	0	10 20 30	40 50 60	70 80 90	100
HOW I FELT *AFTER* EXERCISE					
My mood was:	0	10 20 30	40 50 60	70 80 90	100
My thoughts were:	0	10 20 30	40 50 60	70 80 90	100
My energy level was:	0	10 20 30	40 50 60	70 80 90	100

What I have learned from this:

Seeing the difference between the before and after ratings tells me that:

_____

_____

_____

_____

_____

Which friends? A workout is a chance to experience whatever you choose for a half hour. What should be present during that time to increase your quality of life? Is it the audio book? Is it a radio podcast? Don't rely on exercise alone for entertainment; rely on your ability to add to your exercise experience. Running in time to a song can help you experience your music differently, and, by downloading your favorite radio program from the web, you can have it all to yourself during exercise. (Do, however, take care when wearing headphones. Avoid dangerous situations, because the sounds of passing cars, bikes, and rollerbladers can be blocked by loud music. Try exercising with just one earphone in place, to keep yourself appropriately alert when exercising outside.)

PLANNING YOUR ROUTINE

As you plan your exercise routine, we want you to attend to two criteria: ease and joy. By ease, we are referring to the degree of difficulty you will have getting yourself to show up for your exercise session. By joy . . . well, that is obvious, isn't it? We want your exercise sessions to be as joyful as possible. Think about what you will wear, what you might listen to, who you want to be with, and what you want to see.

What to Wear?

Cinderella might have said, "The right pair of shoes can change your life."[9] If you run, your shoes will be an important part of your routine. Go to a sports store and ask for help; pay special attention to the degree of arch support and the sturdiness of the shoe. Also, the right clothes can enhance your workout experience. Protect yourself from being too hot or too cold. With practice, you will become adept at layering your clothes during cold-weather outdoor exercise. (New wick-dry fabrics can keep you more comfortable in hot or cold weather; being dry keeps you comfortable and reduces chafing. The only limitation to wick-dry clothing is that they tend to wick body odor as well. Don't leave used wick-dry exercise clothing in a heap at the end of the workout—the degree of odor can surprise you.)

Who to Exercise With?

Exercise partners are an excellent way to avoid relying on your own motivational efforts. While you may not show up by yourself at the gym for a workout on a given day, you will probably show up to avoid disappointing a friend. This is the value of a team—having others depending on you and making you feel part of a greater good. Review your friends. Who might join you for a workout? How can you use a friend as a motivator for at least one workout a week? How can you use a shared sport activity to make a workout feel effortless? Exercise partners also make exercise time social time—see if you can use your exercise time to have more time with a valued friend or partner.

Where to Go?

If you have selected an outdoor activity like running, biking, roller-blading, jogging, or walking, selecting your route beforehand may help you mentally prepare for your exercise. Also, using distance markers (such as intersections, businesses, or schools) to help you break up your activity into smaller parts can keep your workout interesting. See if you can characterize each part by a feelings state (hard, easy, full of struggle, coasting), so that you can feel the transitions that your natural terrain offers. Also, be aware of the challenge of your warm-up period. The first section of your exercise may be the most difficult. It is here that your motivation may wane, before you have a chance to get into the swing of things. Remind yourself that you may be particularly stiff or tight, and that you may be especially out of breath as you first get your body moving. Assume the start may be challenging, and wait for your exercise to get better as you get into the flow of things.

Also, think of your route as a form of tourism. What do you want to see? What do you want to experience? How can you maximize your sense of play? Does cutting across the local track help you feel faster? Does running on a path feel better than on the sidewalk? Running is an excellent way to get to know a new city. If you travel for work, consider running or walking in the city you're visiting (check with the hotel for recommended routes and for safety concerns). You will get to know the city better, and you will return from your trip with valuable memories from *outside the hotel* to mark your visit.

Finally, remember that the Internet provides resources for outside exercisers. See the Appendix for examples.

Perspectives from Champions

I like to break up a workout (or a long set) into smaller, more manageable chunks. I often tell myself, "You're on the downhill side" when I get halfway, and this makes the workout seem shorter.

John Naber, 1976 Olympics, Gold (4) and
Silver Medalist – Swimming

Tracking Your Distance or Your Heart Rate

Tracking your runs can help them feel more interesting and can give you goals for specific workouts. Simple-to-use and inexpensive pedometers and heart rate monitors allow you to assess your exercise distance or intensity. You can also use them to check your dose of exercise, as discussed in Chapter 7.

EXPECTATIONS FOR SUCCESS

Your exercise is for you and for your mood. It is a chance to approach the world with appropriate selfishness—doing what you need to do to feel better today. Keep this in mind as you think about your next workout. You are doing it to feel less stressed, less down, and

---

Perspectives from Champions

Once I commit to going to the workout, I'm going to complete it no matter what. I am a strict trainer and follow a regimen, which is how I've always trained. I use music now but never did when I was active because that technology hadn't been developed yet (iPods, portable disc players, etc.). But I tended to get myself into a "trance" when I trained, so those props weren't really necessary at the time. I like the diversion that music affords me now though.

Dwight Stones, 1972, 1976, 1984 Olympics,
Bronze Medalist (2) – High Jump

---

more relaxed. You are doing it for the sense of energy it provides and for the sense of being in tune with your body. And, in giving yourself this benefit, take some time to think about how you can make your exercise as fun as possible. As you keep exercising, you will get better at making exercise a rewarding experience. And those feelings of reward will make it easier to stay involved in your exercise program.[10] The key is getting out there and making your exercise a regular part of your life.

[7]

THE EXERCISE PRESCRIPTION

This chapter is devoted to the characteristics of your actual exercise routine. For that, you should consider your level of fitness, the type of exercise you might enjoy, the appropriate starting point for that exercise, and the intensity and duration that you want to target. The goal is exercise success over the long run, so that you can enjoy the mood effects of exercise over time. Start easy and plan well.

DETERMINING READINESS FOR EXERCISE

Your first step in considering an exercise program is ensuring that you are healthy and ready for exercise. Certain health conditions require that you use caution with exertion; for some conditions, exercise requires supervision by a medical professional or is simply not safe.[1] We suggest that you first complete the Physical Activity Readiness Questionnaire (PAR-Q[2]; see Appendix). As the PAR-Q indicates, use common sense when you answer these questions, and keep this questionnaire in your files, so that you can measure readiness on an ongoing basis. We believe that it is always best to be conservative when it comes to your health, and we recommend that you discuss the initiation of an exercise program with your primary care physician. Your health care provider may complete a physical exam and check your blood pressure, weight, and cholesterol levels, and based on these results, she may suggest that you complete an exercise stress test. This may seem cumbersome, but knowing whether you are indeed ready to begin an exercise program on your own is important.

As an additional consideration, a number of people like to use the information gathered during the medical clearance process as motivation to maintain or continue their exercise habit, with the additional goal of achieving meaningful improvements in physical fitness. These individuals have used indicators of physical health—blood pressure, weight, cholesterol, and particularly the good cholesterol or high-density lipoprotein (HDL) levels—to track their improvement in fitness over time. Thus, you may consider having some of these assessments completed again after a few months of exercise to complement the positive feedback from mood benefits with improvements in physical health.

DETERMINING ACTIVITY

One of the next choices you face when starting an exercise program is selecting an activity. Several questions can guide you in this process. What do I like? What do my friends like? What activity can easily fit into my schedule? In answering these questions, you may come up with more than one activity. You may decide that you will join your friend's spinning class on Thursday evenings, and that you will walk or jog around the neighborhood before work on Mondays, and again during the day on Saturday. Spend some time developing a list of possible activities.

As we discuss in Chapter 10, for many people, maintaining an exercise habit requires diversity in activities. Having a list of activities ready now can help you later on. For example, have you ever considered racquetball, cross-country skiing, softball, flag football, kickball, rock climbing, rollerblading or ice-skating, orienteering, or aerobic dancing, boot camp, or cardioboxing classes? All of these involve aerobic activity, but are not as repetitive in nature as running on a treadmill or other gym-like exercises. In addition to these suggestions, in the Appendix, we list links to websites that provide overviews of different activities categorized by intensity levels. These resources are also available on the website http://www.exercise4mood.com.

Accessibility is also an important consideration. The easier it is to get to your preferred activity, the harder it is to be derailed along the way. However, accessibility should not be your only consideration. Consider the example of Lindsey. Lindsey is a 35-year-old single woman with a long history of depression and anxiety. She remembers first being troubled by feelings of anxiety when she was 9 years old. Her family had just moved to a new city so that her father could start a new job. A new city meant a new school and new people. She felt self-conscious the first day of school—a feeling that only became stronger over the years. High school and college were characterized by social isolation. On a daily basis, Lindsey was consumed by concerns about inferiority and inadequacy, leading her to spend much of her free time alone and to choose a career path involving solitary activities because it made her feel "safe."

When Lindsey came to our clinic for help, she expressed an interest in exercise, mostly because she was also interested in improving her physical appearance. She indicated that she had a treadmill at home and that her sister had some free weights that she could borrow. As her therapist, I suggested that she consider a team sport. The rationale was that exercising in a group setting could offer benefits beyond those to be expected from exercising alone at home. Being around other people would provide the opportunity to learn more about her perceptions of herself. Feedback from teammates during and after games would help challenge the image she had of herself as being inadequate and inferior, thereby enhancing self-esteem and mood. Also, being a member of a team would counter-act isolation. The result was that Lindsey joined a co-ed city soccer league that involved games on Sundays and practice on Wednesday and Friday evenings. The prospect of joining the team was daunting for Lindsey, but she decided to choose this as an investment in her future (a payment of anxiety now, for the benefits of better mood and less isolation later). The investment paid off. It did not take long for Lindsey to report the expected benefits: better mood, a better sense of self, and a sense of team that extended to time spent social-izing with other soccer players.

When considering team activities, we recommend that you take into account the intensity of exercise; moderate-intensity and vigorous-intensity activities are more suitable for achieving mood improvement as compared to light-intensity activities. What this means is that joining an eight-member volleyball team, although perhaps ideal for combating feelings of isolation, may not help you as much in terms of the needed mood lift as a pick-up basketball game that keeps you continually active.

When thinking about exercises, also consider *calisthenics*, which refers to a group of exercises that are rhythmical in nature, such as lunges, jumping jacks, sit-ups, push-ups, crunches, and squats. Calisthenics are the main focus of sessions with personal trainers, as well as of aerobic fitness programs or the so-called *boot camp programs* that have become increasingly popular over the past few years. If not done with others, calisthenics can easily be accomplished at home when weather or other considerations push you toward an easy-to-arrange or indoor workout. Consider the following case example.

Gerald was the 47-year-old father of three teenage girls. Depressed mood had never been an issue for him, until about 5 years ago.

Gerald said, "I think it was because life became more demanding." Gerald married his wife in his late 20s and became a father at 31. An accountant at a national firm, he was able to provide for his family and afford a comfortable lifestyle. All three of Gerald's daughters attended private school. The result was increasing financial pressure; his salary increases did not keep up with his increasing financial demands. Difficulty sleeping was followed by lower energy, as well as by increasing feelings of indifference. When his doctor suggested that he was depressed, Gerald started taking an antidepressant. He had been fairly consistent in taking his medication, but found that it had not helped a great deal to improve his symptoms of depression. He also believed that the medication was in part responsible for the 40 pounds he had gained over the past few years.

Gerald had never liked exercise. He had tried running numerous times (often at the suggestion of his wife, who was an avid runner), but could never stick with it for more than 2 weeks. So, when introduced to using exercise to overcome depression, his initial reaction was negative. He had never heard of calisthenics though and was intrigued, especially when he learned that it involved *interval training*—short exercises followed by longer exercises, all varying in intensity. He joined a local fitness club and started going three times per week. The workouts were challenging, but fun. Gerald was surprised to see exercise as something that he could actually look forward to. He was able to make exercise a part of his weekly routine, and, over the course a few months, saw a sharp improvement in his mood.

DETERMINING INTENSITY

In addition to personal preference, activities can be rated on intensity. Intensity is based on how physical activity influences your heart rate and breathing, and can be rated on a range from light to moderate to vigorous. There are several ways to measure intensity. The easiest way is to do the talk test.[3] Basically, if you can talk but not sing during an activity, you are doing moderate-intensity exercise. If you are not able to say more than a few words without pausing for a breath, you are doing vigorous-intensity exercise. A more accurate method involves the use of a heart rate monitor. These monitors are relatively inexpensive devices that are easy to use and provide you with immediate feedback on your intensity during your exercise. They are available at many athletic stores or on the Internet.

How do you interpret the feedback? The heart rate that corresponds with moderate-intensity exercise is between 64% and 76% of the age-adjusted maximum heart rate, where maximum heart rate (HR_{max}) can be calculated by subtracting your age from 220. Exercise intensity becomes vigorous when your heart rate ranges between 77% and 93% of your HR_{max}. The table below gives ranges in heartbeats per minute for both moderate-intensity and vigorous-intensity exercise by age. You can visit http://www.exercise4mood.com to calculate your exact target heart rate.

Metabolic equivalency tasks (METs) are another index for exercise intensity. Without getting too technical, METs express the energy costs of activities, where 1 MET is the metabolic rate of quiet rest (i.e., sitting). Activities can range from 1 MET (sitting) to 18 METs (running at a speed of 11 miles per hour or 5½-minute miles). Moderate-intensity activities range between 3 and 5.9 METs, and vigorous-intensity activities are 6 METs or more. Notice that, as compared to % HR_{max}, METs do not take into account personal variables; it is an absolute as opposed to a relative measure of intensity. This makes it a little easier to help you determine whether you are working at the right intensity. Indeed, you will not need a heart rate monitor; you can simply look it up. More detailed information is provided at

Table 7.1. Determining your target heart rate

Age	Moderate-intensity Exercise 64%–76% of HR_{max} (220 – age)		Vigorous-intensity Exercise 77%–93% of HR_{max} (220 – age)	
	Lower-end	Upper-end	Lower-end	Upper-end
20	128	152	154	186
23	126	150	152	183
26	124	147	149	180
29	122	145	147	178
32	120	143	145	175
35	118	141	142	172
38	116	138	140	169
41	115	136	138	166
44	113	134	136	164
47	111	131	133	161
50	109	129	131	158
53	107	127	129	155
56	105	125	126	153
59	103	122	124	150
62	101	120	122	147
65	99	118	119	144

relevant websites: http://www.exercise4mood.com or http://prevention.sph.sc.edu/tools/docs/documents_compendium.pdf. Below, we provide examples as guidelines.

You may have heard that vigorous-intensity exercise is best for you. This appears to be true for enhancing physical fitness.[4] However, most goals, including improving mood and well-being, can be reached by engaging in moderate-intensity exercise or a combination of moderate- and vigorous-intensity exercise. After reviewing studies on the effects of exercise for depressed mood,[5] we believe that the best information on a full dose is provided by the U.S. Department of

Table 7.2. Exercise intensity determined by metabolic equivalency tasks (METs)

Moderate-intensity exercise 3-5.9 METs	Vigorous-intensity exercise ≥6 METs
☐ Walking at 3–4 mph	☐ Jogging or running at >4.5 mph
☐ Bicycling on flat ground at 10–12 mph	☐ Bicycling on flat ground at >12 mph
☐ Swimming leisurely	☐ Swimming; moderate/hard
☐ Volleyball (noncompetitive)	☐ Cross-country skiing >2.5 mph
☐ Doubles tennis	☐ Singles tennis
☐ Shooting baskets	☐ Rollerblading
☐ Dancing (ballet, tap, modern)	☐ Dancing (step aerobics)
☐ Kayaking	☐ Soccer game

Health and Human Services.[6] According to their guidelines, a full dose of health-giving aerobic exercise is:

- Moderate-intensity aerobic exercise for at least 150 minutes (2 hours and 30 minutes) each week, or
- Vigorous-intensity aerobic exercise for at least 75 minutes (1 hour and 15 minutes) each week.

Another way of looking at this is that you want to accumulate between 500 and 1,000 MET minutes per week.[7] For example, at 3.8 METs (moderate intensity), brisk walking can help you meet your activity goals if you do it for 150 minutes per week ($150 \times 3.8 = 570$). Similarly, two 1-hour rock-climbing sessions (vigorous intensity; 8.0 METs) would also get you there, as it would yield 960 METs (i.e., $120 \times 8.0 = 960$). Or, you could combine different activities. Let's say, for example, you kayaked on Mondays for 45 minutes (45×5 METs = 225 MET minutes), did a aerobics dance class on Thursdays for 50 minutes (50×6.5 METs = 325 MET minutes), and played doubles tennis for 1 hour on Saturdays (60×5 METs = 300 MET minutes). You would accumulate 850 MET minutes over the week and meet your activity goal. If you prefer these exact calculations, our website http://www.exercise4mood.com provides a calculator to help you determine whether you are meeting the activity guidelines.

INITIATING EXERCISE

Following the guidelines from the American College of Sports Medicine,[8] we recommend that you choose a starting point that will allow you to stay with your exercise habit over the long run.

No starting level is too low; success early on is critical to sticking with exercise over time. The key is to start with an activity that allows you to feel good during the activity. As you get used to regular exercise, you can always push yourself more over time. There is also plenty of research suggesting that having a buddy can be tremendously helpful when you are making changes in health habits, like exercise. So, if you are not in shape at present, consider starting with short walks several times a week. Meet a friend at the park, or walk around the block with your neighbor. The goal is to complete what you set out to do. Then, over the course of several weeks, you will notice that these activities become less physically demanding. Then you can consider an increase in exercise intensity. Start small, and make your habit strong.

On the following page is a sample schedule for the initial weeks of an exercise program for a new exerciser. As you can see, the intensity, duration, and frequency of exercise increases over time, taking 3 or 4 weeks to get the activity schedule up to the recommended dose. Of course, you can decide to use a different schedule to get you to your correct exercise dose. The Appendix provides templates that you may use for this purpose.

LOGGING EXERCISE

A specific action plan, with which you set specific, reasonable, and written weekly goals, can help you work toward success.[9] We emphasize *reasonable* because of the importance of meeting initial goals whenever you start something new. Successfully meeting these goals increases your confidence and the overall success of the exercise program.[10] After writing out your goals (consider a simple calendar, see next page), post these goals in a visible location. Again, when

Box 7.1. MY EXERCISE SCHEDULE

Sunday	Monday	Tuesday	Wednesday	Thursday	Friday	Saturday
						1
						12:00 P.M.– walk 1 mile
2	3	4	5	6	7	8
	6:30 P.M. - walk 1 mile					
9	10	11	12	13	14	15
	6:30 P.M.– walk 2 miles			12:00 P.M.– swimming		12:00 P.M.– jog 1 mile
16	17	18	19	20	21	22
	6:30 P.M.– jog 1 mile	6:30 P.M.– jog 1 mile		12:00 P.M.– swimming		12:00 P.M.– spin class

(Continued)

			Box 7.1. *(Continued)*			
Sunday	*Monday*	*Tuesday*	*Wednesday*	*Thursday*	*Friday*	*Saturday*
23	34	35	26	27	28	29
	6:30 P.M.– jog 1.5 miles	6:30 P.M.– jog 1.5 miles		12:00 P.M.– swimming		12:00 P.M.– spin class

you share your goals with others, it is likely you will try harder to meet them.[11]

As you continue with your exercise beyond the first few weeks, decide whether continuing a written schedule of exercise (as well as logging your progress; see Chapter 9) is valuable. There is good evidence that such logging can help people adhere better to their own

---

Perspectives from Champions

I keep a training journal, where I write down all my workouts: split times, heart rates, and how I felt that day. It gives me a sense of accomplishment to see the workout written down on paper, and it also allows me to track my progress. There's nothing more motivating than seeing steady improvements. And, when I don't improve, it helps to have a record so I can figure out why.

Caryn Parmentier Davies 2004 & 2008 Olympics,
Gold and Silver Medalist – Rowing

exercise program.[12] Nonetheless, the people we work with are split on this topic. Some embrace formal logging, keeping a schedule/diary of their exercise progress over time. On the other hand, for some, logging seems to induce flashbacks of homework assignments from school, with all the urges to avoid it. We can respect this, so we only ask that you at least try scheduling and logging in the beginning of your program. Some commercial diaries are sold for this purpose, with spaces for recording the distances and quality of runs, for example. Over time, you can decide to which camp you belong (love or hate logging), and whether to continue logging over the long run.

NOW TO DO IT!

This chapter offered help with some of the technical aspects of your exercise routine: the what, the where, and the how fast. We encourage you to start easy and to plan well, finding an exercise that interests you and best fits into your schedule, one that allows you to step slowly into the habit of regular exercise. Now that you have a sense of what you are going to do, and how hard you are going to do it, it is time to consider how to make that experience as pleasant as possible. That is the topic of the next chapter.

[8]

ENJOYING YOURSELF
DURING EXERCISE

This chapter focuses on ways to approach exercise with as much joy as possible, including strategies to minimize pain as well as to enhance pleasure during exercise. But no matter what you do, your enjoyment of exercise episodes will vary. You will have transcendent exercise sessions, and you will have exercise sessions when your arms and legs feel like lead and you have to push yourself through every step. The good news is that, regardless of how the exercise session feels, you still can get positive mood benefits in the hours after exercise, including the next day. You may seriously dislike an individual exercise session, but you'll still get all the mood gains from it.

Nonetheless, we would like to give you some strategies for finding the most pleasure during your exercise episodes. This pleasure depends largely on how you direct your attention during exercise, and your ability to drink in the pleasures that exercise has to offer. The strategies here are meant to help you learn how to do just that. We want you to get as much pleasure as possible *during* exercise while you await the greater mood benefits that *follow* exercise.

TRAINING YOUR EFFORT MUSCLE

During any exercise, you are eventually going to find yourself at a point of strain and effort, when you will need to decide how hard to push forward. In a run, it may be at the next hill, the next mile, or the next step. In a spinning class, it may be the last 10 minutes, when you are asked to put your stationary bike in the highest gear. At that point, you feel the dull pain of exertion, accompanied by odd feelings in your stomach, chest, or legs. Do you continue, do you try harder, do you pick up the pace, or do you decrease your effort? In deciding whether to press forward, you will be deciding how much to use your *effort muscle* (remember the effort muscle from Chapter 4?). The effort muscle is different from any of your other muscles. It is linked to physical effort, but it relies on emotion rather than the oxygen and glucose required by your other muscles. The effort muscle, as we define it, is a type of self-control effort—an emotional push to get something done. As it relates to exercise, it is the willingness to bear down and try harder. Depending on your exercise, it is used to get yourself to the point of starting your exercise routine, to increase exertion, or simply to work harder, putting up with all the symptoms of exertion and fatigue, so that you can maintain your pace. In essence, it is that part of you that tells you, "Yes, this is hard, but deep down I know that it will bring something very good, so be persistent."

You can see the benefits of having a strong effort muscle. Obviously, it is nice to be able to use it during exercise, but a strong effort muscle also offers advantages in all sorts of areas of your life, and it can affect your overall well-being as well. Luckily, you can strengthen your effort muscle, and exercise can help. Much as we have illustrated in previous chapters, strengthening skills merely takes practice, patience, and a willingness to believe that the change

Table 8.1. Changes in emotional effort

Rate emotional effort (how much you had to push yourself when you confronted the situation) over time using the following 0 to 10 scale:
0 – Easy/No Problem; 5 – Moderately Hard; 10 – Big Time Hard
Record the date of the situation, and see if stress coping shifts over time with your exercise program.

Stressful Situation #1	Date :	Date :	Date :
_____	Rating:	Rating:	Rating:
Stressful Situation #2	Date :	Date :	Date :
_____	Rating:	Rating:	Rating:
Stressful Situation #3	Date :	Date :	Date :
_____	Rating:	Rating:	Rating:

---

will then only be a matter of time. To help you take this leap of faith ("You are telling me this, but I am not sure"), you may consider tracking the strength of your effort muscle over the course of the next few months. Select one or two situations in your life that you find particularly challenging, in that they take a lot of emotional effort to complete. Each time you deal with that situation, simply write down a few notes on how taxing it was. We predict that you will see an improvement as you start using exercise more effectively, and we want you to be aware of that improvement.

Effort Muscles of All Kinds

Olympic athletes are extraordinary individuals, not purely for their athletic abilities, but also for their extraordinary effort muscles.

Perspectives from Champions

For the past 20 years, I have worked out regularly, 5 or 6 days a week. During peak training, this included three workouts a day. I can remember a few workouts where I couldn't wait to get to it, but most of my workouts (we're talking thousands) involved having to push myself, at least a little bit, to get going. But it is always worth it when I finish.

Whitney Post, 1995 World Champion,
2000 Olympic Team – Rowing

Their ability to push themselves to get to workouts, to strive throughout workouts, and to achieve in competitions is amazing. They also get the benefit of habit, and the benefit of knowing that their effort leads to rewards—Olympic-level rewards. Nonetheless, this habit is built upon hundreds and hundreds of hours of exercise, perhaps including multiple strenuous workouts a day. And, during each of these workouts, unlike those of us who exercise for mood, these athletes push themselves to exhausting limits. Yet, even at these extreme levels of work and achievement, you will recognize in their voices some of the same challenges and triumphs that you will face as you exercise for mood benefits, rather than performance benefits.

To provide a complementary perspective, in the accompanying box is an account of using the effort muscle; this is someone who is not working at a championship level, but is simply exercising for mood. The exercise starts when their effort muscle was already fatigued. The goal wasn't performance; the goal was simply making it through the workout to the mood benefits waiting on the other side.

Box 8.1. AUTHOR PERSPECTIVE: EFFORT ALL GONE

I just had the most pathetic run of my life, at least in terms of actual athleticism. My pace reminded me of those comedy sketches, where they put two people in front of a blue screen and have them pretend to jog while a neighborhood view is presented on a screen behind them. They jog in place, up and down, while the projection gives them the appearance of progressing forward. Doing this, I am sure they would have passed me. I was running that slowly: jogging up and down, barely making any movement forward.

It was my first run after a big stressor—my son had been in intensive care after a sudden and severe illness. He had recovered, and was home and safe. The stress was over, I had given myself a full night's sleep, but I was emotionally exhausted. I had not worked out for 3 days, and I had developed lower back pain, the combination of stress and a long flight home—a trip cut short to see my son. I did not feel like running, but thought it would help me transition out of feelings of emotional exhaustion. My first steps felt bad, and the next few steps felt even worse. I made a deal with myself to run at least 5 minutes, and then decide what to do.

At the 5-minute mark, I was willing to keep going, and my back had loosened up some. But I was still slow, and felt like I was carrying an extra 50 pounds. I searched for good music on my iPod, and found myself hating every song. I kept running. At the 20-minute mark, I found one good song. I kept slogging forward. I finished 15 minutes later, still going slowly.

After the run, I stopped in a park to stretch. I did not feel good; but I had sweated, I had moved, and I had time outside. I felt different. I felt like something had changed. I was tired, but in a different way than before the run. I felt more engaged, and relieved. Walking home, I let my shoulders drop. I let my arms swing comfortably. By evening, I felt the stress of the illness being replaced by the joy of my son's improvement. I had perspective.

COACHING DURING TRAINING: REPLACING *OR* WITH *AND*

Training your effort muscle helps you get used to persisting even when tired. When you use your effort muscle, you may feel yourself bearing down as you try harder. Instead of following this natural tendency to bear down, we would like you to use your effort muscle while trying to stay as light and open as possible. No need to grimace when you use your effort muscle. In fact, right in the middle of your exertion would be an excellent time to relax your brow, and try to make an effort be as *open and light* as possible. This is easier than you might think, as long as you are willing to let go of some preconceived notions. Are you used to thinking of effort as the opposite of relaxed? That you are either exerting yourself *or* you are relaxed? But do these categories have to be mutually exclusive? Can you exert yourself in a relaxed way?

In considering these questions, it is helpful to remember that seemingly opposite emotions can co-exist side by side. In fact, many aspects of life can be made more difficult by considering emotional events as mutually exclusive. Consider the following:

- I can be mad at my spouse OR I can have a good relationship.
- I feel really disappointed at work OR I can be in the right job for me.

Now look at the same statements where AND is used instead of OR.

- I can be mad at my spouse AND I can have a good relationship.
- I feel really disappointed at work AND I can be in the right job for me.

If every anger and disappointment nullifies the positive aspects of your life situation, then you can't help but be on an emotional roller-coaster with every stressor. That, or you have to deny half your experience ("No, why would you think I am bothered at work, my job is a good fit for me" and "Oh, I am not mad, I love my husband"). Holding an OR perspective denies the complexity of life; ORs instead of ANDs make life both harder and more inaccurate. Consider the ORs in the realm of exercise:

- I can feel really tired OR I can have a good workout.
- I can be really straining OR I can enjoy the benefits of running.

Each describes a worldview that is more difficult, because choices are limited. Now consider the AND perspective:

- I can feel really tired AND I can have a good workout.
- I can be really straining AND I can enjoy the benefits of running.

Exercise is an excellent way to train yourself to be able to experience the ANDs in life. Your task is to develop a frame of mind that most allows you to enjoy exercise, even with the experience of exertion or fatigue. This is what we mean by open and light—open to embracing the good parts of the experience and in finding joy, even when other parts of the experience are taxing. By not joining with the most negative parts of your exercise experience, and instead dropping your shoulders, relaxing your brow, and relaxing with your exertion, you will indeed feel lighter in what you do.

BE THE DIRECTOR OF YOUR FEELINGS

During the effort of exercise, what is your facial expression? Is your forehead smooth, or are your brows drawn in concerned concentration? Do you have an easy half smile on your face, or do you have a tight-lipped grimace? Check your face, and reset it into the smooth-browed half smile. Then, notice whether your pace changes, whether you have an easier time with the effort you are exerting. If you do notice a difference, your experience is consistent with research on the effects of facial expressions on mood.

A smiling facial expression makes it easier to experience positive emotions; a frown does the opposite. This is true even when a smiling expression is produced falsely.[1] For example, if you watch a cartoon while holding a pen in your mouth in a way that mimics a smile (see Figure 8.1), you are likely to be more amused than if you watched it without this forced expression (that is, if you held the pen in your hand).[1] This suggests that subtle changes you make in your posture and facial expression send messages to your brain about how you feel.[2] The implication is clear: Instead of letting your

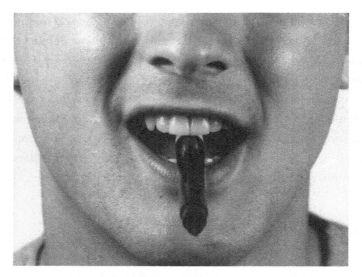

Figure 8.1. Poised Smile (Holding a Pen) Used to Change Mood.
From Strack, F., Martin, L., & Stepper, S. (1988). Inhibiting and facilitating conditions of the human smile: A non-obtrusive test of the facial feedback hypothesis. *Journal of Personality and Social Psychology, 54*(5), p. 771, reprinted with permission.

posture and facial expressions *follow* your feelings, use your posture and facial expressions to *direct* your feelings.

Try out the half smile and relaxed forehead (you may want to check your expression in the mirror before you exercise), and see if it doesn't lead to a better experience while you run—and afterward. And, don't limit this positive action to your exercise session. Start thinking about what you can do differently to improve your mood and anxiety in other situations. The best guide here is to ask yourself, "What would I do if I felt good?" For many people, the answer would be, "My posture would be relaxed, I would be engaged, and pay attention to what is going on right here in the moment." These are all behaviors that are within your control.

MINDFUL EXERCISE

Exercising with a half smile on your face provides some good initial training in mindfulness. By *mindfulness*, we mean a curious attention to the present moment, in an open, nonjudgmental, and accepting manner.[3] Curiosity refers to the frame of mind by which you approach your experience. Instead of knowing how you should interpret the next event or the next sensation, thought, or emotion you notice, with mindfulness you approach that event with curiosity: a "Hmm, let me check out what I am feeling," rather than an "Ugh, I hate feeling sweaty."

You can hear the absence of judgment with the "hmm" approach. This is an important aspect of mindfulness. Rather than immediately categorizing your experience as good or bad (with an "Ugh," for example), in mindfulness you approach the next event or sensation with open-eyed curiosity ("At this moment of my life, what does it really feel like to be sweaty?"). Without immediate categorization (good or bad, tolerable or not, etc.), many sensations and experiences are much more tolerable than we would otherwise assume.

It is this process of conceptually sitting back and observing your emotions that describes the concept of mindfulness. Mindfulness includes not only a sense of detachment from a single provocation, but the ability to be aware of multiple inputs at any one time, and to decide which input should get your attention.

Think about your experience right now as you read this book. You are absorbing the content of what you are reading, you feel the pages on your fingertips, and you are aware of the amount of light and noise in the place where you are reading. You may also be aware of your breathing rate, a bodily discomfort, or the feeling of your shoes on your feet. Mindfulness refers to the ability to be aware of these many inputs, without being automatically captured by one.

And, if you are not captured by one, you have the freedom to shift your attention to more fully experience a different input. Shift your attention to what it feels like to hold this book. Are the pages warm or cold? How smooth do the pages feel against your fingertips? How comfortably can you hold the book? What memories does the feel of the paper bring? This is an example of mindfully experiencing a single input: helping yourself curiously notice the experience and drink it in more fully. This is an ability we would like you to practice during exercise: Be aware of physical sensations or emotions during exercise, but don't be overly captured by them.

But to take that moment to find out how tolerable a sensation actually is, you will need a way to inhibit your immediate and automatic judgment. To make yourself stop and not follow your habit, we recommend *marveling*. We introduced you to marveling in Chapter 5, when we were discussing reactions to thoughts. We asked you to marvel at your thought content, to buy yourself time to evaluate the thought, rather than simply reacting to it emotionally or behaviorally. As part of mindfulness, we want you to expand your marveling skill to help you examine your reactions to sensations and emotions, rather than just your thoughts. Marvel at the way in which you are coaching yourself, "Wow, check out what I am saying to myself," and marvel at your physical experience as well, "Wow, check out my reaction to sweating."

Your job is to be amazed by and curious about how you react to sensations, to communicate to yourself a sense of wonder and interest. Why wonder? Because there are a lot of ways to react to sensations like sweating, breathlessness, fatigue, and the like. Chances are you have fallen into a rut across your lifespan, choosing to react in one particular way. Marveling gives you a chance to develop a new way of reacting. The goal is to have a fresh experience of the sensation by noticing what it *actually feels like*, instead of what you *think it should feel like*. And, in fully noticing the sensation, the task is to see if you can react to the sensation in a way that gives you more pleasure and less distress.

Getting the Most Out of Marveling: Relationships

As an aside, you should know that marveling works well in relationship conflicts. Conflicts in romantic relationships happen so often because we care so much, and because we have so much time to develop biases in how we think. We have all sorts of ideas about what our partners are thinking or doing, and we are really ready to categorize ("He said that because he thinks I . . ."). With these categories in place, it is easy to react emotionally in ways that we may later regret. Marveling at times of relationship conflict buys you time and provides you with a way to more calmly react to provocations of the moment. Instead of reacting automatically ("I can't believe she said that"), take a moment to marvel at the experience. In terms of your self-coaching, it may sound like this:

> She did say that, and, wow, I really have an urge to get mad. In fact, look how hurt I am and how ready I am to react with an angry retort. First, I am going to marvel for a moment at the strength of my emotion . . . then, second, I am going to decide what sort of response best serves me and my relationship.

As you can tell, marveling is a good strategy for avoiding getting automatically hooked into an emotional response to a provocation.

BEING IN THE MOMENT: PRACTICING MINDFUL THOUGHTS

Mindfulness helps you to be able to run when fatigued, for example, without counting every step. Mindfulness helps you to have the thought of quitting early, but to decide to find a feeling of comfortable relaxation in the fatigue. Mindfulness helps you to listen intently to your music while also breathing hard and thinking about your running route. Mindfulness training also helps you to not take your thoughts too seriously. It helps you to notice your sensations, your emotions, your thoughts, and your exterior environments as an ongoing stream of information; it is up to you to decide what to pay attention to. To develop this ability, practice directing your attention with open curiosity to the wealth of your current experiences. Here is a four-step example for practicing this process during aerobic exercise:

1. Start by noticing where your attention is directed (is it on your breathing, your fatigue, your movements?). Let's assume you are paying attention to your feelings of fatigue. Now notice what you are thinking to yourself about your fatigue (this is your interpretation of your feelings). Notice that your interpretation of your fatigue is different from the fatigue itself (notice, for example, that your actual feeling of being tired is different from your tendency to say "This feels lousy").

2. Consider your fatigue and your thoughts about fatigue as two different events. Let yourself be very curious about each event. Then, practice shifting your attention between the two: Think really hard "this feels lousy" for 10 seconds, then notice what your fatigue actually feels like for 10 seconds. Do all this while you continue your exercise, so that your attention is flowing

between the thinking, feeling, and moving parts of the exercise experience. These are three different events.

3. Now, rather than focusing all your attention on feelings of fatigue or your thoughts about fatigue, shift your attention to something more fun (e.g., the look of the trees if you are outside, or the feel of the water on your arms if you are swimming). Notice how you feel while shifting this attention. Now, play around with shifting your attention between the trees (for example), your thoughts about fatigue, and your actual feelings of fatigue.

4. Now, pick the attentional focus that is most pleasurable, and let the other topics float to the background. Continue to exercise, but let your facial expression reflect what you are devoting your attention to.

This is where the half smile comes in. A half smile is a reminder that your mood does not have to be owned by the most aversive aspects of your experience. Take running for example. Let's assume you are running on what appears to be a "bad day." You were tired at

---

Perspectives from Champions

It is getting the workout started that is the hardest for me. After a good warm up, the middle of the workout is the best part. The middle of the workout puts me into a Zen. I can think and find solutions to problems; it is a time to unclutter my brain. Trying to set a base time/distance to improve on is always good for me, though, I do not set my goals too high.

Daniel K. Sayner 1980 Olympic Rowing
(USA boycott)

the start of your exercise, and you are tired now. You are aware of every step; in fact, you are counting every step, and grimacing while you do so. Then you remember the half smile. The half smile helps you remember to be open to lots of inputs at the same time, and to choose which inputs and which responses help you the most. Counting steps: not helpful. Grimacing: not helpful. Setting a half smile, noticing the trees and the sky, and settling into a better day-dream while you extend effort: helpful. Marveling at your habits, reminding yourself to be curious and open to the entire range of your experiences, and spreading your attention out more evenly—that is mindfulness.

LESS WORRY, MORE PROBLEM SOLVING

One terrific benefit of an exercise session is that it is makes it hard to worry. Many people report a decrease in ruminative (repetitive) thoughts while they exercise. For your authors, it takes at least 20 minutes of exercise for ruminations to quiet. Then, whatever repetitive thoughts that have been with us throughout the day start to lose their salience. A calm, quiet mind emerges.

You can help this process by not overfocusing on worries. Chronic worry patterns are characterized by a tendency to actively restart worries. It is like sticking your tongue in an empty tooth socket; it hurts, but it feels irresistible. And, even when you force your tongue to the other side of your mouth, it is only a matter of time before it comes back searching—checking to see if it still hurts.

In the most common worry pattern, people bring up a worry, focus on it for a while, and then jump to a new worry. This process soon acquires a life of its own, and it becomes easy for worries to cycle around in a nonstop fashion. This is when a reset button is needed—a way to stop this cycle and clear the head. Exercise can provide this, but the exerciser needs to be ready to embrace this change, to not restart the worries when a moment of respite comes. For this reason, we want you to be prepared to look for, enjoy, and embrace a shift in thoughts when it comes. Rather than restarting a worry, take active pleasure in the shift in focus ("Ahh, now I am less connected to that thought") and take the opportunity to refocus your attention on something more pleasant (your music, the feel of your body, the sunlight through the trees).

This does not mean that we want you to use exercise to ignore important problems or feelings. The art of being mindful is in finding the right level of attention to problems and emotions—it is as important not to underfocus on issues as it is not to overfocus. One way to help ensure that you are not ignoring important issues is to schedule weekly problem solving sessions with yourself (as discussed in detail in Chapter 5).

To sum up, using exercise to deal with worries is a two-step process. First, use exercise to break up ruminative thinking, and use mindfulness to embrace the quiet mind that exercise brings. Second, ensure that problems do get your full attention with a clear mind. Set up focused, weekly problem solving time, with a pen and paper at hand to help define problems that need solutions.

PLAYING WITH PACE: TAKING THE ANXIETY OUT OF SENSATIONS

Moderate to moderate-strong levels of effort and exertion are as hard as you ever need to push yourself to enjoy both the mental health and physical health benefits of exercise.[4] Nonetheless, many readers may want to choose more taxing exercise regimens as part of other fitness goals, or as part of athletic competitions. Also, more taxing exercise provides a way to get used to some of the bothersome sensations that play a role in anxiety disorders.

As discussed in Chapter 2, panic disorder is one of the anxiety conditions that can be helped by exercise. Panic disorder is an anxiety condition characterized by recurrent panic attacks. These attacks are sudden rushes of anxiety symptoms—for example, a pounding heart, breathlessness, dizziness, numbness and tingling sensations, chest pressure, or choking sensations—that seem to come out of the blue. These sensations can feel overwhelming to panic sufferers, and they are often interpreted not as anxiety symptoms but as signs of a catastrophe—things that are frightening in their own right— like a heart attack, stroke, or nervous breakdown. In fact, it is the fear of these symptoms that helps keep panic disorder alive.

Below is a figure illustrating a core intervention used in the cognitive-behavioral treatment of panic disorder. It involves the step-by-step presentation of symptoms similar to the feared symptoms of a panic attack. Patients are shown how to recreate these symptoms with simple exercises (e.g., running in place), and they are given a chance to get comfortable with these sensations. In fact, patients are asked to practice inducing the sensations between sessions, trying not only to decrease their fear of sensations like dizziness or a rapid heart rate, but to get bored by these sensations (moving from an "uh oh" response to a "relax with it" response). As patients achieve this comfort level, the panic cycle ends. Figure 8.2 illustrates this process of inducing feared sensations, noticing them, and relaxing *with* them, while practicing doing nothing to control them. This last part is important. By just letting the sensations be there, individuals have a chance to learn to react differently (nondefensively) to their bodily sensations. When people stop desperately trying to stop the sensation, the body calms down and fear subsides.

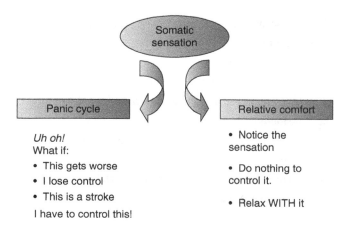

Figure 8.2. Reacting differently to feared sensations.
From Otto, M. W., & Smits, J. A. J. (2009). *Exercise for mood and anxiety disorders* (Workbook).
New York: Oxford University Press, reprinted with permission.

As you can tell, intentional exposure to feared bodily sensations makes use of mindfulness skills: noticing a sensation (like a pounding heart) without being captured by automatic reactions to that sensation (such as, "Uh oh, I have to make it stop"). As you might has guessed, exercise as a way to expose people to feared sensations can be used successfully as a treatment for panic disorder.[5] Fears of anxiety sensations (anxiety sensitivity) decrease with programmed bouts of exercise. Hence, if you are suffering from panic disorder, or just find sensations of emotional arousal bothersome, then you will want to apply mindfulness to both the sensations of exertion and the thoughts that accompany these sensations. Here is one way we have directed patients undergoing panic treatment:

As you increase the intensity of your exercise (as your fitness increases), part of the goal will be to exercise vigorously enough to produce bodily sensations similar to those you experience during a panic attack. Prior to and during this vigorous exercise, you will want to:

1. Remind yourself of what sensations you are going to feel so that there are no surprises (e.g., dizziness, rapid heart rate, light-headedness).
2. Complete the exercise, fully expecting to experience these sensations.
3. Notice the sensations and see how comfortable you can get with exercising while having the sensations.

After you complete the exercise, try not to wait for the sensations to go away. Just become good at tolerating them. Remind yourself that it does not matter how long these sensations last because they are not dangerous (given that your physician has approved your exercise); therefore, you don't have to get rid of these sensations.[6]

To help you become more comfortable with bodily sensations of exertion, approach your exercise as if you are playing with feelings of exertion. Changing your effort during exercise, such as increasing your pace during running, gives you a chance to see how different levels of exertion feel, and a chance to become comfortable with these sensations.

To help yourself attend mindfully to sensations of exertion during exercise, consider keeping a log of your experiences during vigorous exercise (see Figure 8.3). This log provides you with a way to track the sensations you experience, rating their intensity on a 0 to 100 scale, and examining how these sensations impact your emotion. Also, we want you to be aware of the negative interpretations

---

Date of Exercise:_____

What sensations did you experience during your exercise?

_____

_____

How intense were the sensations during your workout (0–100)?

Beginning :

Half-way :

Toward the end :

What was your anxiety level throughout the session (0–100)?

Beginning :

Half-way :

Toward the end :

What were the actual consequences of the sensations that you experienced, particularly when you tried a mindful perspective on these sensations?

_____

_____

How did these consequences differ from any specific fears you had about these sensations or urges you had to control the sensations?

_____

_____

What do you want to tell yourself about these sensations now?

_____

_____

_____

Figure 8.3. Exercise Practice Log for Panic-related Concerns.

From Otto, M. W., & Smits, J. A. J. (2009). *Exercise for mood and anxiety disorders* (Workbook, p. 73). New York: Oxford University Press, reprinted with permission.

of these sensations that increase anxiety. Like other anxiety-provoking thoughts, these thoughts are usually about future events and take the form of, "What if . . . ?":

- What if these sensations get worse?
- What if I lose control?
- What if something is wrong with me?

These thoughts are classic in panic disorder, and all have a role in transforming natural sensations into fearsome events. The exercise log provides a space for you to examine whether these thoughts are accurate. Was there any actual danger associated with these sensations, or was it okay just to note them mindfully and to continue with your exercise? The information you put in the log will guide you in your next exercise session. More information on panic disorder and its treatment can also be found at relevant websites (see the Appendix).

ENHANCING PLEASURE

If nothing else, exercise provides you with a break from your regular routine and the opportunity to find unexpected riches. It provides you with moments to attend to new aspects of the world, to be with different people, to experience novel things. Even with something relatively repetitive like running or swimming, exercise gives you a chance to enjoy sensations for sensation's sake. The feel of a breeze against your skin while running deserves to be noticed and enjoyed mindfully. Likewise, the feel of water on your body and the sounds of your breathing deserve mindful attention while swimming. Outdoor activities put you in closer contact with the environment and the seasons than you might otherwise be: the feel of light rain, the shift in scents as autumn comes, the difference between your cold face and warm body in winter, and the first springtime experience that nature's first green really is gold.[7] Part of the benefit of exercise is getting practice in being vigilant to what is good and pleasurable.

And, when you are just too tired for this vigilance, then it is time for good music, a good book, or good television during exercise. Exercise machines at the gym or at home lend themselves well to these pursuits. We have friends who get their week's academic reading done during exercise, and we have friends who watch their

> **Perspectives from Champions**
>
> Lately, I've been reading my law school textbooks on the exercise bike. I have to do the reading anyway, so I might as well kill two birds with one stone and get in a workout at the same time. It takes some practice to be able to concentrate on what I'm reading, but I find in the end that I remember the material better that way.
> Caryn Parmentier Davies 2004 & 2008 Olympics,
> Gold and Silver Medalist – Rowing

favorite recorded television shows or movies while on the home exercise machine.

The key is approaching exercise while being prepared to be entertained by at least a part of the experience. The process of mindfully shifting your attention among inputs may offer you mood benefits, in addition to the mood lift that exercise itself will bring you. Shifting attention in this way may well strengthen the part of your brain that acts to dampen down the ruminations that occur during depression. Shifting attention also makes you able to enjoy richer experiences. You can't lose—whether it is a useful brain exercise for fighting the ruminations of depression or simply a way to drink in joy while exerting yourself, guiding your attention mindfully has its benefits. Figure 8.4 provides five ways to try to enhance your mindfulness during exercise. We picked items that can be done while running outside. We picked running because it is an exercise open to almost everyone and because running can be very monotonous if you do not use strategies to drink in joy. All of these activities assume that you have a safe area in which to run, and that you are not prone to tripping or running off the road while playing around with your attention.

Table 8.2. Mindful running exercises

- Look at a tree intently. How would you draw or paint it? What colors are in the bark? How many colors other than green are in the leaves? How does this tree differ from a prototype tree? How does it move in the wind?
- Notice the breeze against your forearm, first on your left side, then on your right side. How would you describe the feeling? What is pleasant about it? How central can you make the feeling to your awareness?
- Of all your senses, how can you make music more central over the next 3 minutes? Instead of passively listening to the music, let yourself fall fully into the tones. How does your sense of the world change as the music takes over?
- How are you holding your arms and shoulders? Can you help them relax, dropping your shoulders and letting your arms swing more freely as you run? Notice how your hands feel. Are they wet? Are they comfortable? Touch your fingers together on your right hand. What is pleasant about that? Continue your run while trying to let your hands enjoy the experience.
- Every minute or so, make sure you breathe in through your nose. Notice what smells you can identify. Notice subtle differences in the scents. Marvel at how many scents you miss because your attention is elsewhere.

LOOKING FORWARD TO THE MOOD SHIFT

Mindfulness is useful for helping you direct your attention toward joyful moments during exercise, and not letting you become overly distracted by ongoing discomforts. Many feelings of discomfort occur early in exercise, before you and your body get into the swing of things. Warming up slowly can minimize these feelings, but probably will not eliminate them. Knowing that your attention can be fluid, and knowing that you can enjoy pleasant moments despite uncomfortable feelings, will help keep your motivation up during your first 5 minutes of exercise. It is also useful to remind yourself of the benefits to come. Clear expectations of a mood lift after exercise make it easier to invest in the drudgery of the first few minutes of exercise. Blind faith—knowing that it will get easier as you go along and that you will enjoy mood benefits when you are done—is a great antidote to those first few minutes of "ugh." Remind yourself that exercise is your break, a chance to clear your head and reset your mood. Look forward to what you will experience during your exercise session, so that you can take your mindfulness—a curious, open, and nonjudgmental attitude—with you, helping you be ready to enjoy whatever comes next.

Fact or Fiction?: The Runner's High

As the popularity of running sharply increased in the 1970s and researchers discovered natural opiate-like compounds in the brain (known as *endorphins*), the experience referred to as "runner's high" attracted widespread attention. Nonetheless, difficulty in defining and measuring this subjective experience has led to controversy over whether a runner's high actually exists.[8] Those who have attempted to define the term emphasize two components: (1) feelings of euphoria and (2) enhanced insensitivity to pain. Anecdotal accounts, however, are widely available and varied. Some describe short periods characterized by intense joy, peace, and energy. Others describe milder feelings of well-being, while still others deny experiencing such feelings.

The feelings of transcendence or joy that get labeled a "runner's high" are not specific to running. Any exercise that offers prolonged exertion brings with it the potential for these feelings. How much exertion is needed is not known. Early research suggested that at least one continuous hour of aerobic exercise was necessary, but even this idea has come into doubt, with some evidence for similar physiological changes brought by shorter bouts of exercise.[9] And the physiological basis for this experience? There is some evidence that these feelings are indeed due to activity of endorphins, but even that evidence is far from certain. Given the elusive nature of a runner's high, we don't want you spending your exercise time searching for one, but we do want you to emphasize you mindfulness during exercise—this will put you in a great position for enjoying feelings of transcendence should they occur.

A RICHER EXERCISE EXPERIENCE

This chapter was designed to change the way you approach your exercise experience, while you are in it. This will take some practice, and it may be helpful to reread this chapter prior to a number of your workouts, so that you are prepared to think about how you are using your effort, where you are directing your attention, and whether you can adopt a more mindful and open approach to your exercise experience. In doing all of this, try to retain a curious attitude, asking yourself how you can best use a half smile during your next workout. And don't forget to apply the same principles to fully enjoying the warm shower afterward!

[9]

REWARDING YOURSELF
AFTER EXERCISE

The moment you finish a workout, reward yourself after exercise with two immediate lines of thought. First, say to yourself something like, "I did it, another workout in the bank." Second, allow yourself a satisfied smile. Both the statement and the smile are an accurate acknowledgment of the investment you just made in your well-being. You got yourself to your workout. You put in the time. And, fast or slow, smooth or rough, light or heavy, fleet-of-foot or trudging, you finished. This is what you need to attend to as part of your mood management: the completion of regular workouts of moderate to high intensity.

Giving yourself credit and enjoying the effects of your workout are the topics of this chapter. We need to take time to cover these topics because so many people have trouble giving themselves credit. This difficulty can stand in the way of both enjoying and extending your exercise achievements.

How well do you give yourself credit? If you are like many people, the answer is "Not very well." Across life, it becomes easy to devote attention to what is *not* working rather than what *is* working. On any given day, when you have down-time moments—at a stop light, while in an elevator, while in a checkout line—what do you think about? Are you reliving every low point of your day? Are you reviewing problems? Or, are you giving yourself a chance to notice what is working well in your life, what is good, and how you can have more of it?

WATERING THE FLOWERS, NOT THE WEEDS

Problems deserve your attention; this is why we encourage a formal problem solving approach in Chapter 5. But your achievements deserve at least equal time. By focusing on what is working, as well as what is not working, you have a better chance of making the most of your successful moments.

Think of it in terms of gardening: We want you to water the flowers, not the weeds. During down-time moments—the elevator, stop light, checkout line, etc.—review your daily successes and what led to them. We think of this process as *echoing* the good moments in life. Just like an echo, you get to have multiple reverberations of a positive event. Instead of having a pleasant moment occur only once, we want you to make sure it occurs once in life and then several more times in memory.

ECHOING EXERCISE

Speaking of echoing, try echoing your exercise successes across the day. This includes not only a repetition of the "I did it" phrase, but also a review of what was most positive about your exercise, and how it made (and is making) you feel. And don't be afraid of attending directly to feelings of fatigue or soreness that you may be

Perspectives from Champions

My reward for a workout is getting a shower and feeling good about myself for the rest of the day.

Gary W. Hall, MD, 1968, 1972, & 1976 Olympics, Silver (2) and Bronze Medalist – Swimming

experiencing after exercise. These feelings are markers of your achievement. Fatigue says that you treated your body well, using it and making it appropriately tired. Muscle aches are likewise a marker of strong workouts. Don't be shy about seeing a physician if discomfort is strong or persists. But otherwise, feelings of muscle recovery are to be celebrated for the fitness and mood effects they reflect.

Echoing exercise successes can also help maintain your motivation for the next exercise session. These periods of review help keep the role of exercise in mood management clear, and help keep exercise appropriately high in your hierarchy of motivations (see Chapter 4). When echoing exercise, make sure to review all the positive aspects of the experience. You will have some days of clear achievement in which, for example, you biked or swam farther or better than you expected. But, on many days, the echoing experience might be around something you saw, felt, or thought about during your exercise. Also, as part of tracking your ability to be mindful during exercise, think specifically about how you changed your attention during exercise, and whether you had moments of adopting the curious attention to experience that we discussed in the last chapter.

In addition to reviewing positive moments during exercise, also take time to review positive changes that occur after exercise. Is your mood different? How about your reaction to stress? Is there a change in your sense of energy or your sense of engagement in your surroundings? Has your sleep quality changed? Knowing how exercise is serving you will help you keep up with your regular program of mood and stress management.

Consider extending echoing to sharing your experiences with your support team as well. The more you verbalize and share your achievements and associated mood and benefits, the better off you are in terms of establishing a durable physical activity habit. This is exactly the reason why some people love to keep an exercise log. It isn't just about recording the exercise, but about marking achievements and the joyful aspects of the exercise experience (see p.209).

PROBLEMS WITH COACHING

If you are exercising for relief of depression, be especially vigilant to how you are coaching yourself after exercise. The voice of depression is focused on watering the weeds. Moods actively color our memories and our perceptions. When you feel down, you will naturally remember other times when you were sad. This is because your mood is acting as a memory cue. Just as the smell of cafeteria food may remind you of being in grade school, a negative mood will bring to mind past times when you were sad. In this way, your failure experiences crowd your internal experience, making it hard to see all the ways that things are working well for you. Feeling down also influences you to devote more attention to bad things and to ignore good things that are going on currently.[1] In the morning, at the mirror, you will notice your skin blemishes instead of your eyes; at work, you will notice your coworker's silence rather than her nodding approval; and when it comes to exercise, you will notice when your work out went poorly rather than when it went well.

When you are in a low mood, actively counter these tendencies. Do not let them get past you unnoticed! Ensure that you focus on the pleasant moments of exercise. The more negative your mood, the more important it is to actively echo and to actively coach yourself around your successes. To give you a sense of what this may be like, we have included an example. In our clinical work, we are face to face with mood biases on a daily basis, and our job is to help our patients see their achievements more clearly. In the following dialogue,[2] we have captured this experience in the interactions between a therapist (T) and patient (P).

T: As you settle into your exercise program, I would like you to pay extra attention to how you are talking to yourself about your experience of exercise. Your motivation for exercise, and the degree to which you enjoy your exercise and post-exercise experience, may depend on how you direct your attention and how you coach yourself. For example, I want to make sure you are paying attention to the achievements you have made so far in adopting an exercise program. You have been exercising for 3 weeks so far and have succeeded in exercising two to three times per week. Have you commended yourself for these efforts?

P: Well, not really. I mean I missed two exercise sessions.

T: You did miss two sessions, but you made seven sessions. This effort deserves some notice!

P: I guess I have done okay.

T: I want you to be careful about how little credit you give yourself. If you heard that a friend started an exercise program and made seven of nine scheduled sessions, what would you say?

P: I guess I would say "good job," especially if they are just starting out . . . like I am.

T: Good point—someone starting out with a new program deserves encouragement. And since you are the coach of yourself in this effort, it will be important for you to commend yourself for your efforts.

P: Yeah, I guess so.

T: So, let me hear it. Have you been on track—do you deserve a "good job"?

P: Yeah. Good job for me [smiles].

T: Nice. [pause] And while we are on the topic of coaching yourself, have you noticed what you tend to think about during exercise?

P: Oh, yeah, I noticed that sometimes when I run I tend to count my breaths. It gets really tedious.

T: I bet. If you find that you are counting your breaths, what might be more interesting to direct your attention toward?

P: I guess what is going on. In fact, I was running alongside a park the other day, and I noticed this tree that was changing colors. It was beautiful, and I noticed that I don't often pay attention to that sort of thing in the city. Sometimes, my wife and I will drive out in the country to see the leaves, but I don't even notice them very well when they are on a tree just down the block. But on my run, I did happen to notice the colors.

T: It sounds like you have one alternative to counting. If you notice that your attention has fallen to something boring on your run, you can redirect yourself to see if there is anything interesting to look at along the way.

P: Yeah.

T: And, how about after your runs? How do you tend to feel?

P: You know, I feel tired, but I usually feel good. I am not sure I am getting much of a mood lift in general, but after the runs I feel peaceful-like. I feel tired but good.

T: I like that phrase, "tired but good." I think the phrase captures a reality about a type of mood shift that happens from exercise. Exercise does make you physically tired but emotionally refreshed. I think "tired but good" captures that shift in mood.

P: Yeah, it is kind of neat to feel that. I usually just feel tired, or tired and cranky, at the end of the day.

T: As part of coaching yourself effectively around your new exercise habit, I want you to make sure to reflect on this "tired but good" feeling and remind yourself that you are changing your mood with exercise. You have farther to go in the exercise program before we expect bigger changes in mood, but if you attend to, remind yourself about, and make sure to enjoy the mood changes you have had so far, it will help you maintain your motivation for the next exercise session.

P: That makes sense; sounds good!

Keep in mind that you will have to play the role of the therapeutic coach, using the same voice you use when giving advice to people who are important to you. If you get someone else to help as well, that is great. But you are the main coach. It is up to you to provide yourself with a guiding voice that gives you credit for what you have done.

LEARNING FROM YOUR EXPERIENCES

An additional part of self-coaching is planning well for your next exercise session. Given how your last several bouts of exercise have gone, how do you want to direct your attention during exercise? Do you need different music? Do you need different clothes? Is there a friend you now want to involve in exercise? Also note what helps you get to your exercise sessions, particularly when your motivation is low. Keeping a regular log of your exercise program can help you in this process. Surprisingly, just keeping a log will enhance your ability to stay with your exercise.[3] For any sort of log, start by finding yourself a notebook, something that you find pleasant enough to keep handy on your desk. For a weekly log, we recommend keeping track of the date and type of workout, a rating of the intensity of the exercise, and then writing about what was noteworthy or most pleasant about the exercise. To make things easy for you, an example log form is available in the Appendix and on our website at http://www.exercise4mood.com.

TRACKING YOUR MOOD CHANGES

In addition to attending to the mood benefits of individual exercise sessions, try to track how your fuller program of exercise is benefitting your mood. In the Appendix, we provide you with a copy of the Quick Inventory of Depressive Symptomatology (QIDS)[4] as a way of assessing depression severity. We recommend you repeat your QIDS assessment every week, to regularly assess how your exercise program is working for you. We expect your depression to decrease across weeks of exercise, but, in the treatment of depression, individual profiles of improvement differ. Some individuals report the same score for weeks and then suddenly experience large gains in 1 week; others may have slower and steadier improvement over time. And, it is possible that you may have difficulty improving from exercise. If this is the case—that you are not improving despite regular exercise across weeks of training—do not hesitate to seek additional help. The Appendix provides you with resources for finding this additional help. But do continue your exercise; used alone or in combination with other strategies, exercise can improve well-being in a multitude of ways.

COMPENSATORY EATING AND SITTING

We prefer to focus on the active positive—what to do, rather than what not to do. Nonetheless, there are two activities that deserve caution: compensatory eating and compensatory sitting. *Compensatory eating*—when people increase their food consumption after exercise—has been shown to nullify some of the expected weight-loss benefits of exercise programs.[5] Be particularly vigilant of the tendency to use food as a reward for exercise. By this, we don't just mean the classic vision of a person jogging to their local coffee shop for a donut, but the more subtle decisions of how you load up your plate during your meals, or whether you select an extra dessert during the day because you have exercised.

We also want you to be wary of *compensatory sitting*—the tendency to sit more during the day because you have exercised. For some, additional sitting is seen as a reward for exercise ("I ran this morning, I might as well take it easy now"); for others, it may be a reaction to feeling fatigued ("I should relax to recover"). As we explain below, there are excellent reasons—whether you are tired or not, happy or not, busy or not—to break up your sitting times and to reduce the overall time in which you are sedentary, independent of how much you exercise. However, before we get to strategies for minimizing compensatory behaviors, it is important to review the nature and scope of health behavior compensation, starting with eating.

The Notion of Compensation

There's a widespread belief that healthy eating cancels out unhealthy eating. And by belief, we don't mean that people carefully think through and decide that healthy food cancels out unhealthy food, but rather that most people have an automatic (and illogical) assumption that it does. Here is the evidence. Researchers had two groups of adults, 934 in total, look at pictures of high-calorie food—things like a meatball pepperoni cheese-steak, a bowl of chili, or a bacon-and-cheese waffle sandwich. One group saw one of these items presented alone. The other group saw one of these items presented with a healthy side dish—a small green salad, celery and carrots, etc. Both groups were asked to estimate the total calories of the food they saw. Not only did the adults who saw the high-calorie food plus the side dish fail to increase their calorie estimates (it is a larger meal, after all), but they gave *lower estimates* of the total calorie count. It is almost as if they expected the carrots and celery to vacuum calories out of the cheese-steak. As the author of the study comments, "People behave as though healthy foods—such as fruits and vegetables—have 'halos' that extend to all aspects of the meal, including its effect on weight gain."[6] Of even more concern is the finding that this halo effect is stronger in those individuals most concerned with weight loss.

This halo effect is one explanation for the failure of many weight loss attempts. The shift to a diet cola will not remove the calories from a double cheeseburger, and the fruit smoothie at McDonalds will not improve health if it provides a green light for ordering a Big Mac. Similarly, exercise will not improve the waistline if it gives us permission for an extra donut and whipped cream caramel coffee.

To help you avoid compensatory eating, make sure you are fully attentive to the rewards of exercise. The adoption of healthy behaviors should never come at the expense of joy—but that joy, and any rewards you may want to give yourself, doesn't need to come from the realm of food. As you well know, one central and powerful reward for exercise is the reduction in stress and improvement in mood. No need to compensate for that. Exercise gave you a better mood; it is already a fair deal! But if you want more rewards, think of other things you may want to give yourself. Table 9.1 provides a list of common, pleasant events, those events that give people moments of pleasure and are generally inexpensive. If you need a reward, consider selecting one from the list instead of choosing something from the pantry.

Compensatory Sitting and . . . Death!

With a dramatic heading like that, we had better explain. It is clear that exercise, in addition to helping you feel happier, less depressed, and less stressed, will also help you live longer. In addition to these powerful effects from formal periods of aerobic exercise, general activity levels are also key. In particular, it is important to avoid prolonged sedentary (primarily sitting) time. Here is the evidence. In a recent, large-scale study, prediction of death rates were examined

Table 9.1. Pleasant event list

- Walk outside and look at the sky
- Take a bath with candles around the tub
- Reread a book you read in high school or college
- Sit on a porch swing
- Write a letter to a friend
- Do a crossword puzzle (each day for a week)
- Take a kid to mini golf
- Call two friends and go bowling
- Climb a tree
- Put on some music and dance in your living room
- Go for an evening drive
- Sing a song
- Have a tea party on your front porch
- Meditate
- Paint (oils, acrylics, watercolor)
- Read the newspaper in a coffee shop
- Buy flowers for the house
- Listen to your favorite song from high school ... really loudly
- Play with a Frisbee
- Rent a video and invite friends over

Table 9.1. (Continued)

- Plan a garage sale (perhaps with a neighbor)

- Walk in the snow and listen to your footsteps

- Buy a spool of wire, and make a sculpture

- Take a really long shower

- Read a novel

- Play a video game

- Buy a magazine on a topic you know nothing about

- Get a massage

- Polish your favorite shoes

- Find your top three favorite videos on You Tube and share them with a friend

- Buy a new plant

- Write poetry

- Do Sudoku puzzles

- Plan a poker night

- Go to an art museum and find one piece you really like

- Sit in the sun

- Clean out a closet

- Burn a CD of your favorite movie music

- Repaint a table or a shelf

(Continued)

Table 9.1. (Continued)

- Play a musical instrument

- Start a scrapbook

- Play with children

- Plan a hike for the weekend

- Start writing a journal

- Have a picnic at a park with a friend

- Go bird/nature watching

- Read a book under a tree

- Organize photos/CD collection

- Visit a pet shop and look at the animals

- Plan to go fishing in a local stream or pond

- Catch snowflakes in your mouth

- Invite friends over for board games

- Learn to knit

- Plan a garden

- Volunteer to walk dogs for a local animal shelter

- Plan an affordable 3-day vacation

- Start a collection of heart-shaped rocks

- Plan a drive in the country

- Learn to fold dollar bills into origami creatures

Table 9.1. (Continued)

- Soak your feet in warm water
- Learn to juggle
- Clean and polish the inside of your car
- Organize a weekly game of cribbage or bridge
- Read about places you've always wanted to visit (and maybe plan a visit!)
- Go to the beach
- Take a photo (every day for a week)
- Go to the zoo
- Play horseshoes
- Go to a sporting event
- Attend a local art event (a dance performance, a play, an art show opening)
- Lie by a pool/river/lake/beach
- Join a museum Friday night event
- Take a yoga class
- Take a historic tour of your city

Table adapted from Otto, M. W., & Smits, J. A. J. (2009). *Exercise for mood and anxiety disorders* (Workbook). New York: Oxford University Press.

over time in 53,000 healthy (disease-free) men and over 69,000 healthy women. Across the 14 years of study, there were nearly 19,000 deaths in this group. Independent of the level of exercise, the time spent sitting was associated with death. Those who sat more than 6 hours a day, compared to those who sat fewer than 3 hours a day, had a 34% increased risk of death![7] This association was strongest for cardiovascular disease deaths. When risk of death was examined for people who tended to sit for prolonged periods as well as engage in adequate exercise levels (as recommended in this book), the risk of death was almost double for women and one and a half times for men, as compared to those who did not sit for long periods and who did exercise. In another study, a link between two specific sedentary behaviors (riding in a car and watching TV) and cardiovascular death was found for a large sample of men studied for more than 21 years.[8] Normal weight and greater physical activity offered protective effects for these men.

Aside from reducing the total time spent sitting, adding in breaks during sitting time may be important for maintaining health. In a study of 168 people who provided[9] detailed information on sitting and activity over a week-long period, a break in sitting time was linked to a number of important health outcomes ranging from waist circumference to triglyceride levels and plasma glucose, all factors that are linked to the development of diabetes and other health conditions. In this study, a break in sitting time was defined as at least 1 minute of increased activity (such as standing up and walking or pacing briefly). Why might this movement be helpful? As you might guess, it is in the way the skeletal muscles utilize energy; they are a major clearance site for glucose and plasma triglycerides. That, and moving around helps increase total daily energy use. These study findings were powerful enough for us, your authors, to adopt two strategies during the prolonged desk time it took to write this book. First, we worked hard to remember to stand and either pace or stretch at the end of each hour of writing. Fortunately, our academic schedules are such that such prolonged writing time is unlikely to be found during the day, but at night, prolonged writing is possible. So, we stood and paced. But, in addition, between the writing of individual paragraphs, we adopted a policy of exaggerated fidgets. These fidgets involved leg lifts while sitting (extending each leg several times while at the desk) as well as arm upward stretches.

We recommend similar activity for you during your daytime or nighttime television, driving, reading, or desk time. In addition to standing up and walking between television shows, for example, we recommend leg lifts, arm lifts, or presses at every commercial break.[10] Figure 9.1 summarizes this movement. It is important to remember that these mild exercises are not an alternative to the aerobic exercise that we encourage in this book; these small breaks are a separate life-saving effort to reduce the ill-effects of prolonged sitting. No matter how much you exercise, these breaks from sitting are important. And, by the way, regular fidgeting does burn calories, especially fidgeting done while standing and walking, providing another strategy for managing the energy balance required to maintain a healthy weight.[11]

Also, look for alternatives to prolonged sittings. At the many scientific meetings we attend, it is not unusual for the program to involve 8 to 10 hours of sitting across the day. But we don't sit. During periods of the meeting, you will find us standing at the back or side of the room. With years of this practice, we can assure you, it is not rude or overly distracting to the speakers. Indeed, the most frequent comment we have received from other attendees is the stated wish that they had stood more (to reduce back pain, bottom pain, or to keep the meetings more stimulating). So, we encourage you to think about when you can stand and move more: during television time, between or during meetings, or when on the phone.

Finally, we are reminded that Winston Churchill wrote at a standing desk. This idea has been taken one step further with the advent of treadmill workstations. Indeed, a recent *New York Times* article[12] documented the three to six miles a day logged by employees while they typed at their computer screen. Some will even hold meetings while walking backward on their office treadmills. Enthusiasts report that it takes at least as much coordination as walking and chewing gum, but we suspect that more is required. We don't know if this mini-fad will last, but the trend is already marked by its own social network (http://officewalkers.ning.com/). We do like the idea of integrating movement and exercise with desk time, and it is clear that walking and working strategies can provide dramatic increases in calories burned during the day.[13] For us, perhaps a treadmill or standing desk will be on order for our next book.

- Place your hands on the arms of your chair, and complete 5 to 10 press ups (lifting your bottom of the chair seat by straightening your arms). If your arms feel too taxed, you can press up lightly with your legs to make it easier.
- Lift your arms, touching your hands together above your head. Do ten such lifts and touches, slowly.
- Lift one leg at a time, straightening your leg, with your foot off the ground, while staying seated. Do each lift slowly (1–2 seconds lifting, 1–2 seconds returning your foot to the ground), and complete five lifts with each leg.
- Press your heels into the ground (you will feel the backs of your legs and your bottom tighten). Flex this way for 3 seconds, and then relax. Repeat 5 to 10 times.

Figure 9.1. Brief exercises for television commercial breaks.

BRINGING IT ALL TOGETHER

In sum, part of your motivational power comes from giving yourself credit for on-track behaviors. We discussed the importance of echoing these moments across the day, particularly at moments when you might otherwise daydream about worries or concerns. For the next several weeks, practice searching for and echoing the positive daily events that occur. Echoing will make your traffic light, check out line, and elevator time more pleasurable, and will serve as a motivation guide to keep your on-track moments happening. In addition, this is the perfect time in your life to re-evaluate your self-coaching and to use your self-talk to give yourself credit where credit is due. Finally, we introduced the ideas of compensatory eating and sitting. More information on eating patterns and activity levels is provided in Chapter 11, but at this point, consider how you can use exercise as part of more general activity promotion. From the number of times you walk to the water fountain at work, to what you do during television commercial breaks, the present is an excellent time to use activity to help you become generally more active in your daily routine.

[10]

DIVERSIFYING YOUR
EXERCISE ROUTINE

"Ugh, not this again!" As with any activity, you will face the risk that, over time, your exercise routine will start to feel repetitive and dull. Instead of looking forward to your exercise, you may begin to dread it, and your feelings of pleasure will start to be replaced with a sense of irritation. Boredom happens, and we want you to be ready for it. Boredom is not a sign to stop exercise; instead, it should be a sign to *start approaching your exercise differently*.

One key to maintaining a strong exercise habit over time is variety. Variety includes changing exercise habits and context—things like the music, clothes, workout buddies, time of day, and place of your workouts—as well as the type of exercise you complete.

Any single exercise routine has lots of parts. Do you exercise outdoors or indoors, alone or with a friend, with music or without? To what do you pay attention? What are your goals? About what are you daydreaming? All of these factors make a difference in how exercise feels. And how exercise feels makes a difference in how long you will stay with it. As you know, good versus bad feelings during exercise predict whether people stay with or give up on exercise over time.[1] Therefore, be vigilant to what you need. Although occasional boredom is okay, regular feelings of boredom are not. If boredom

Box 10.1. BOREDOM RELIEF PLANNING

- Where have I been exercising? _____

What changes might give me more to look at, experience, hear, or feel during my exercise? _____

- When have I been exercising? _____

What times of day may give me a different motivation to exercise? _____

- What have I been thinking about during exercise?

_____

How can I better direct my thoughts during this time?

_____

- What have I been listening to during exercise?

_____

What might be better ways to make my exercise time interesting?_____

- With whom have I been exercising?

_____

Can I find a better way to make my exercise time feel more social?

_____

- What have I been doing for exercise?

_____

(*Continued*)

Are there ways I can change up this routine to make it more
interesting? _____

- What other types of exercise might I like to try at this point in
  my life? _____

Given this, what is my plan to add more pizzazz into my
exercise? _____

becomes a regular part of your exercise routine, we want you to
intervene actively, starting by asking yourself what contributes to
the boredom that *you* experience during exercise.

NOW THAT I AM BORED, WHAT SHOULD I DO?

Let's discuss some things that you can do during exercise to curb
boredom. In a recent study,[2] researchers asked a group of individuals who were exercising at least an hour a week to try out different
types of imagery during exercise, such as recreating a past exercise
scene that was really enjoyable or imagining the energy they felt in a
previous exercise situation. Here, people were encouraged to think
of sounds, colors, and other elements related to the scene to create a
vivid image. It turns out that imagining enjoyment and energy
helped people feel better during exercise. Those who used these
techniques experienced more positive feelings during exercise and

---

Perspectives from Champions

The idea of being the best is quite motivating for competitive athletes. I used to think about all my competitors and how I would outwork them in training. I would visualize all the time about competing against my biggest rivals during my workouts.

Darrin Steele 1998 & 2002 Olympics – Bobsled

---

felt more revitalized after exercise than did people who exercised without using imagery techniques.

Turning to energetic and enjoyable images during exercise can be complemented or perhaps facilitated by the type of music that you have available on your iPod or other music player. This can mean simply switching from rock to classical, trying the music that your friend recommended, or making exercise the time when you listen to a audio book. The idea of limiting certain music or book listening time just to exercise time can be a powerful influence on helping you get the exercise you need to enhance your weekly well-being. You get book time and you get exercise time, and you get both as long as you are firm with yourself and only listen when you are moving. In addition to helping you combat boredom, music can help you meet your specific exercise goals. In a recent study,[3] recreational bicyclists were assigned exercise while listening to no music, preferred music, or nonpreferred music. As you might expect, listening to preferred music resulted in better performance as rated by perceived exertion and greater riding distances. Nonpreferred music had no benefit, so it is important to choose your music well.

Although changing what you do during exercise is effective, don't hesitate to make a full-scale change in the type of exercise you do.

Perspectives from Champions

I use exercise time as my "creative time" for work. In the midst of the workout, I am thinking about what business problems I need to solve and how I might do it. I definitely use music and if stationary, video.

Olympic Gold Medalist – Men's Rowing

As one of us experienced recently, sometimes it takes a new beginning to keep exercise feeling fresh see Box 10.2.

SEASONAL CHANGES

While a core exercise (e.g., biking, running, or swimming) may carry you through as a regular workout regardless of the time of year, you may want to bring other types of exercise online during those months of the year that best support them. Seasonal team activities can provide motivation to show up, try hard, have fun, and to make use of the fitness you have cultivated during other seasons. Having one workout a week devoted to a novel activity can provide you with some natural cross-training and reward you for the fitness you have achieved.

Also, seasonal changes provide new ways to make your regular exercise interesting. Running in snow is a challenge in its own right. If you try it, remember one of the caveats of ice driving courses (yes, there are ice driving courses over really awesome frozen tracks): You can turn and you can brake, but you can't both turn and brake at the same time. That is, you can't if you want to keep control of your car.

Box 10.2. AUTHOR PERSPECTIVE:
BOREDOM INTERVENTION

My regular exercise had been a four-mile route in my neighborhood, twice a week before work and then once on the weekend. I felt pretty good about the fact that I had been meeting the public physical activity health dose, but had started becoming concerned about keeping it up. Indeed, getting up early every morning to go outside and pound the pavement, facing the same sights (and often the same people on the way) had become merely a demanding task instead of a rewarding activity. Having joined many gyms without actually going in the past, I did not consider this a realistic alternative. I had always enjoyed tennis, but then could not think of this becoming a regular activity. Then, one day, one of my friends suggested I join her in a new workout group. This workout group was organized by professional trainers and offered sessions three times per day on six days of the week. This was not the usual workout; this was something new in that it combined interval training (low-intensity followed by high-intensity exercises), sprint and agility drills, and *plyometrics* (hops, jumps, and bounding movements) all in one session. Other attractive features of this workout were that sessions were always different, the sessions were held at public parks around the city, and the sessions were group-based. I signed up, and almost immediately noticed an important shift: Instead of coming up with reasons not to exercise, I started looking forward to it. Importantly, boredom during exercise was replaced by joy.

(*Continued*)

Why the shift? First, the simple change from just running to interval training combined with exercising other parts of the body such as arms, chest, and abdomen made the workout appear less repetitive. Second, having an instructor telling me what to do and when to do it added an element of surprise, making the workout less predictable and more interesting. Third, working out in a group rather than alone turned exercise into social interaction, and made it a more fulfilling experience.

The same principle applies to running in snow and ice; slow down *before* turning. In fact, slow down generally, and be prepared to use a shorter stride to better keep your feet under your body. If you do so, you may discover that running in snow can be especially joyful: the smell of the air, the softness of falling snow, and the ability to pass cars spinning their way along the street. Making use of seasonal changes is just one way to keep your exercise interesting over the long haul.

TRYING NEW THINGS: BEING GOOD AT BEING BAD

One requirement for joyfully trying something new is that you have to be good at being bad at it. That is, if it is truly new—meaning you are stepping outside your skill and comfort zone—then you need to be prepared to be a beginner. The joy of being a beginner is in the experience, tasting and seeing things that you have never experienced before. Trying to be *good at* this new experience? Why, that is unfair to the whole process!

We believe that, every so often, you should actively seek out something that you are bad at. Doing this provides you with such a clear and palpable reminder that the goal is not perfectionism, the goal is joy. Joy can exist at every stage of competence, as long as you don't take yourself too seriously. And, it may take some good self-coaching on your part. Actively remind yourself that you are a beginner, and take that first yoga, dance, climbing, kung fu, or volleyball class with a smile on your face and a readiness to learn. When you find yourself to be the only one facing the wrong way in class, smile again and learn. And take the lesson with you—it is possible to demand so much of yourself that everything you do feels like a failure. Instead, let yourself learn, and let yourself be happy with far less than perfect. There is more joy at this level.

MIXING IT UP: INTERVAL TRAINING

Recent studies have shown that *interval training* can provide some dramatic benefits compared to continuous moderate exercise.[4] These gains can be achieved in as little as 2 weeks. Interval training alternates sprint-level intensity with recovery periods. The timing of these two periods differs dramatically between studies, with some programs calling for 30-second sprint bouts interchanged with 1 minute recovery periods,[5] and others utilizing 4-minute (bike) sprint periods alternating with 2-minute recovery times.[6] The number of these intervals (sprints and rest cycles) vary, with somewhere between four and ten of each, which means that you can achieve a very intense workout in very little time. Interval training is linked to enhanced muscle and fitness building as well greater fat-burning capacity. As such, it provides a tempting strategy for those who want to get in better shape for competition, as well as for those who want to improve fat burning and other health indices. The only problem with interval training is, well, the intervals. The sprint is hard, admittedly less hard at the 30-second level than the 2-minute duration, but still hard.

During the sprint interval you will be acutely aware of your effort and fading stamina. In fact, one of your authors is certain that during interval training he once passed through Kübler-Ross' emotional stages of dying: you know, Denial, Anger, Bargaining, Depression, and Acceptance.[7] The problem with the intervals is that you get to the rest period before you get to Acceptance. Then you have to start over at Denial ("I can make it, it isn't so hard"). Okay, we are exaggerating, but interval training is a very different workout. This is its value. By shifting to interval training on some of your workouts, you can use these challenges to more quickly change your fitness level as well as change the feel of your longer, slower workouts. With interval training, you can provide yourself with very diverse workouts and make the longer, slower workouts feel easier, a restful break from the high-intensity ones. But make sure you are healthy enough for this training; check with your physician if you consider shifting to these higher-intensity cardiovascular challenges. And don't forget to warm up before and cool down and stretch after interval training.

Perspectives from Champions

I like to be creative with the sets I do and vary my training a lot, so I do something different each time. Once I am in practice, I like to set goal times for myself to make it more challenging.

Gary W. Hall, MD, 1968, 1972, 1976 Olympics,
Silver (2) and Bronze Medalist – Swimming

REMEMBER THAT YOU'RE IN IT
FOR THE MOOD LIFT

Now that we have encouraged you to consider the joys and challenges of high-intensity workouts, we want to caution you about these workouts as well. One of the additive joys of exercise over time is in observing how your body and your abilities change with continued workouts. If you exercise regularly, depending on how you exercise, you will become faster and stronger in what you do, and will have more endurance for future activities. If you combine your workouts with regular stretching, you will find that your body will support you in more activities. Movements will become easier, chronic back pain may decrease, and you may keep your breath in activities that used to tax you. This means you have potential for more fun in more activities.

Increasing fitness may also lead you to increase your performance demands for workouts. This is a natural consequence of improving fitness; you expect a more fit performance. However, we would like you to be very careful about how you coach yourself around these increasing performance expectations. Seek a balance between maximizing performance and achieving optimal mood benefits. In terms of maximizing your mood benefits, remember that any moderately strenuous workout hits the mark. Feel good about it—even hard workouts that you struggle through. Understand that these days are going to happen, and avoid self-criticism. You got out there, you exercised, your body gave you at least part of what you demanded of it, and you put yourself in line for mood benefits. Don't undo these gains by calling yourself names. You need to be ready for and understanding of variable performance. Be firm with yourself, asking yourself for a better workout later in the week, but do not sap the joy from whatever workout you do get.

Perspectives from Champions

A goal such as a race, rowing regatta, or backpacking trip is always good to have and seems to help me make improvements in the quality and quantity of the workouts. Most importantly, it is a healthy behavior adding time on my life.

Daniel K. Sayner 1980 Olympic Rowing
(USA boycott)

We are not saying not to strive to perform well or compete, we just want you to be careful to not let the competition take on a life of its own. We want you to exercise for the joy it brings, so protect at least one preferred exercise from the competition bug!

EXPANDING YOUR EXERCISE TEAM: YOUR FAMILY

In solidifying and diversifying your exercise habits, consider how best to involve your family and friends. Everyone wins if exercise time is occasionally family time—as long as balance between activities is maintained. Having at least one workout a week with a family member or close friend offers the benefit of shared time, shared goals, and the spread of the health benefits of exercise to those you love. You also get the potential benefit of support for your health habits from family. There is always the danger that exercise time detracts from valued family time—motivating a push-back from family—and this is an effect we do not want to see. Making exercise time shared time helps ensure support for your activity, and guarantees that it stays infused within the broader search for joy that we hope is at the base of family time.

For your romantic relationships, you may especially want to consider trying new exercise activities, at least those that are within your current athletic abilities. Karate programs, dance lessons, and rock climbing classes are available in most major cities. Likewise, more atypical activities such as trapeze classes are also becoming increasingly available (talk about an abdominal muscle workout!). If these activities seem daring, it may be just the ticket for your relationship. Some research suggests that arousal upon meeting or interacting with a potential romantic partner, regardless of source (e.g., fear from a swaying bridge to, believe it or not, exercise), can be (mis)attributed to the romantic partner who shared in the activity.[8] It seems there the body gets confused about the source of the excitement, and the excitement is attributed to the romantic partner, as long as that partner is viewed as at least moderately attractive. We assume that this is still the case for your relationship. If so, because of the anxiety and thrill of a shared trapeze class, *you* may be seen as more attractive by your romantic partner. We are not saying that you specifically need to be seen as more exciting and arousing by your partner; we just don't know any couples that can't benefit from this effect. Think about it.

Don't Forget the Kids: The Benefits of Exercise for Youth

The occurrence and emotional cost of depression in children and adolescents is a startling reality. Early episodes of depression are also linked to a recurrence of depression across the lifespan,[9] motivating the need for both early treatment as well as an ongoing mood management strategy. Depression in youth is also linked to a much broader set of health problems. For example, depression during adolescence, at least in girls, is associated with more than a doubling in the likelihood of obesity in adulthood.[10] In these girls, depression often recurs over time, and the risk of obesity is even higher for girls who have had multiple episodes of depression. Part of this effect may be the way in which depression is itself associated with poor eating habits, specifically the eating of fried or processed foods, refined grains, and high-sugar products.[11] Part of this effect may also be due to activity levels and exercise itself. During adolescence, girls often undergo a marked decrease in physical activity,[12] and a depressed mood may decrease this even further, setting off a feed-forward cycle of poor mood, reduced activity, and an even worse mood.

The dramatic rise of childhood obesity in the United States has been well documented.[13] Between 2003 and 2007, obesity rates among U.S. children increased by 10% (18% for girls), with an overall 2007 obesity rate of 16%.[14] Almost one-third of children were overweight at this time period. Rates of obesity were linked to television viewing time and recreational computer use, and, as you might expect, lower levels of physical activity. The health impact of this obesity epidemic is striking, with obesity linked to the development of diabetes and other cardiovascular risk factors, including asthma.[15] Exercise and weight loss provides important protection against this risk, and even at the early age of 5 years, regular physical activity is linked to lower levels of emotional and behavioral problems, in addition to its physical health benefits.[16]

Exercise has other benefits as well. One such benefit appears to be work success. Yes, work success! Here is the evidence. A recent study has shown that people who had been involved in high school athletics have 14% to 19%[17] higher working wages in adulthood. While it is not clear which aspects of athletic involvement help bring about this association, it is clear that it is not simply a difference in education or family background; rather, it may be that athletics helps kids develop skills to increase personal and work productivity in life. Athletes learn how to compete well within the rule structure of a given sport, and also learn how to operate within a team structure to work toward a clear goal. They also learn how to maintain motivation and focus on a goal, despite adversity (the effort muscle). All of these skills may provide benefit in the working world.

Okay, parents, let's review. So far, we have evidence that exercise in youth can help them become healthy and wealthy. How about wise? Yes, wise as well. Research on youth indicates that exercise has benefits to attention and memory,[18] just as it does in adults.[19] As such, exercise can give your child a better opportunity to learn. Whether or not that translates into better grades depends on other factors, like whether that improved learning ability is applied to academic pursuits or just a quicker reaction time for a video game.

Helping Your Child Start an Exercise Habit

You can use both bottom-up and top-down strategies to help your child develop interest in exercise. For the initial engagement of the child's own interests (bottom-up), emphasize exercise in the context of fun games. There is evidence that children find exercise more enjoyable when the focus is not on competition and winning.[20] Instead consider: (1) focusing on participation with family members, with parents encouraging and participating in activities; and (2) providing a broad array of choices, to see what particular sport or activity captures a child's interest. But remember that unstructured activities may be preferred to any structured activities. If a child does try a team sport, keep in mind that mistakes are common. Most children will look to parents when these mistakes occur, so parents have an important role to play in keeping those mistakes in perspective and focusing on the joys of participation.[21] Children have a range of motivations for exercise, including the excitement that they feel when involved in an activity, satisfaction and pleasure from learning a new skill or decreasing a weakness, learning something that may be useful later in life, or simply enjoying the mood benefits.[22] Cultivating an interest in competition and winning can come later.

As a top-down strategy, parents can think about how to involve their children in their own exercise habits. Jogging strollers revolutionized the ability of parents to make exercise time family time, at least for toddlers. In addition to regular family walks, parents can get more aerobic effort by having their children bike or scoot along with them on a safe track or bike lane. Parents should also keep in mind how easy it is to exercise in the context of chase games, or sports (such as a half hour of shooting baskets). These strategies not only help parents, exercise but introduce children to the idea that exercise is a regular part of adult life—an expectation that may help keep the exercise habit alive as your child develops.

As children transition into the teen years, use of exercise for weight management and sculpting of body shape becomes more important, as does the role of social networks within sport teams. Nonetheless, family and peer support, participation, and encouragement can help keep your child motivated to continue to expand his or her aerobic activities (see Appendix for website resources). In all of these exercise promotion activities, start early and keep it fun.

FINDING THE RIGHT BALANCE

Keep in mind that exercise, like anything else, needs balance. Among young women, overexercise can be a symptom of distortions in body image, as well as the reliance on body for self-image. These concerns can strike successful female athletes, where overtraining and under-eating (disordered eating) can shut down the menstrual cycle and place the athlete at serious risk for loss of bone density and other health issues.[23] The body mass index (BMI) tables presented in the next chapter are useful for identifying when weight is falling too low. Likewise, if eating patterns seem unhealthy, then early intervention is in order.[24]

Seeking balance in the frequency and intensity of exercise is part of the overall message of this chapter: diversify your exercise experience to enhance your feelings of well-being. Balance can include drawing on your different levels of expertise—doing things you are good at and making sure to also occasionally introduce new things that you are not good at. As we stated earlier, joy can exist at every stage of competence. The key is not taking yourself too seriously. And, when it comes to exercise, while you are seeking diversity, remember to keep your focus on getting your mood lift and enjoying the process of moving and being fit.

[11]

EXTENDING YOUR ACHIEVEMENTS: AN ACTIVE AND FIT LIFE

The purpose of this book is to guide you in developing and maintaining a regular program of exercise that will help you overcome stress, depression, anxiety, or other mood challenges. Along the way, we have also introduced you to a number of other important principles for managing behavior, including information on the nature of motivation and self-control. We have particularly focused on the importance of arranging your environment, and in chaining together behaviors, to help you feel more like doing the things you care about. In many ways, our maxim was not *more effort*, but *more environment, better thinking, and easier effort.* The goal was to help you learn how to finesse your environment and your habits, so that you rely less on internal self-control efforts.

Now, consider leveraging this training and your exercise successes into making sure you get to enjoy your better mood over the long run. This chapter is dedicated to helping you use your current skills to enhance some of the physical health benefits of exercise.

EXERCISE BENEFITS: WEIGHT LOSS AND OBESITY PREVENTION

If you are exercising regularly, you may already be starting to notice some of the changes in vitality that come with a stronger body. You may find it easier to do things—play with the kids, climb stairs, have endurance at work—and you may feel the sense of body and strength that goes with being more in shape. These are expected changes. Programmed exercise not only improves mood, but increases feelings of vitality, improves physical function, and enhances social functioning.[1] It is now up to you to decide whether you want to add weight loss to this list of achievements. Because you are primarily exercising for your mood and well-being, if you want to lose weight (for either health or appearance reasons), define that weight loss as a separate goal.

Our purpose for this section of the book is to help you use what you learned in previous chapters to better arrange your lifestyle for additional health goals. And, we want you to keep improving your mood while you do so. Before we get to those strategies, let's look at some of the other advantages of exercise, including the benefits of weight loss if you are overweight or obese.

As you know, exercise offers a wide range of health benefits; with increasing cardiovascular fitness, on average you can expect to live longer, regardless of whether you are currently healthy or whether you are recovering from a health condition.[2] Yet, as beneficial as exercise and cardiovascular fitness may be, it is even better when you are at a healthy weight.[3] Maintaining a healthy weight is associated with specific reductions in cardiac risk factors, as well as with reductions in all of the health risks linked to diabetes. Much of the research on the link between weight and morbidity (diseases) and mortality (death) uses accepted definitions of overweight status and obese status. These categories are based on calculations of *body mass*, calculated from height and weight tables, such as the one on page 177 (please visit our website http://www.exercise4mood.com if you want to calculate your exact body mass index [BMI]). The BMI provides an estimate for healthy body proportions based on height and weight, and it is sensitive to the percent of body fat you carry. The BMI is a widely used index for identifying weight problems.

In providing you with this BMI table, we expect a certain amount of surprise about the weight ranges that define overweight or obese status. Along with the increase in weight and obesity among adults and children in the United States, there appears to be a growing acceptance of higher weight standards. It appears that Americans are getting used to the idea of being overweight, and are changing their perspectives on how people should look. That is, ideas about how someone should look depend in part on what people are used to seeing. What you see, in turn, depends on where you live, because obesity is not distributed evenly across the United States. For example, 16.4% of children across the United States were classified as obese as of 2007. However, rates differed dramatically between states, ranging from more than 1 out of 5 children in Mississippi classified as obese to a low of 1 out of 10 children in Oregon.[4]

Some of the state-to-state variation in obesity rates appears to be accounted for by household and neighborhood environment characteristics such as modes of transportation (influencing walking rates, for example), income (influencing the availability of leisure time and/or food choices), safety (keeping kids indoors), limitations on the availability of recreational facilities (opportunity for exercise), or the ready availability of fast-food outlets (ease of high-calorie food choices). But even when factors like these were taken into account, children in Georgia, Kentucky, Tennessee, and West

Table 11.1. Body mass index table

	Normal	Overweight	Obese	Extreme Obesity
BMI range	19–24	25–29	30–39	40–54
Height (inches)	Body Weight (pounds)			
58	91–115	119–138	143–186	191–258
59	94–119	124–143	148–193	198–267
60	97–123	128–148	153–199	204–276
61	100–127	132–153	158–206	211–285
62	104–131	136–158	164–213	218–295
63	107–135	141–163	169–220	225–304
64	110–140	145–169	174–227	232–314
65	114–144	150–174	180–234	240–324
66	118–148	155–179	186–241	237–344
67	121–153	159–185	191–249	255–344
68	125–158	164–190	197–256	262–354
69	128–162	169–196	203–263	270–375
70	132–167	170–202	209–271	278–376
71	136–172	179–208	215–279	286–386
72	140–177	184–213	221–287	294–397
73	144–182	189–219	227–295	302–408
74	148–186	194–225	233–303	311–420
75	152–192	200–232	240–311	319–431
76	156–197	205–238	246–320	328–443

Virginia remained at more than twice the rate of obesity as children in Oregon. How does this happen?

There is evidence that obesity travels through social networks. For example, among adults, the likelihood of being obese is linked to whether a person's family and friends (their social network) are obese.[5] According to population research, the chance of becoming obese increases by 57% if a person has a friend who became obese. In terms of family members, an individual's chance of becoming obese is 37% if he or she has an obese spouse. The chance of obesity was similar (40%) if a person had an obese sibling. As such, it appears that standards for eating, exercise, and appearance may be shared between individuals, as well as in communities, thus influencing the likelihood of obesity.

This is part of the value of the BMI standards; they provide a standard for weight independent of the people we know and the communities in which we live. The standards are reprinted here not to induce shame (shame rarely results in useful behavior), but to identify the health ranges where weight has been associated with poor health outcomes. Our hope is that, if you decide to change your weight-related risk factors, you might also influence your family and friends. It follows that if obesity travels through social networks, expectations for exercise might also spread through these networks. In other words, we hope that exercise and its benefits will be contagious—that over time, your family and friends will *catch* these activities from you. But that is only possible if you take the lead on exercise and weight loss, if this is an appropriate goal for you.

FOOD AND MOOD

In terms of at least one crucial risk factor for weight gain, you have already taken some important steps. A sad, blue, or depressed mood appears to be a powerful motivator for overeating.[6] By getting the mood benefits from exercise, you are reducing the likelihood that you will be in those moods that influence poor eating choices. Also, choosing to do something valuable (exercise) when faced with a bad mood helps you avoid one important weight-gain pattern: eating in response to low moods. Such a dramatic link exists between food and mood that it pays to go through this information more carefully, particularly as it relates to depression.

Depression and eating patterns are clearly linked, including what you eat. For example, in a recent study in the United States, a dietary pattern characterized by vegetables, fruit, meat, fish, and whole grains was associated with a lower likelihood of depression and anxiety disorders. In contrast, a diet characterized by processed or fried foods, refined grains, sugary products, and beer was linked with higher mood distress scores.[7] This study was cross-sectional, meaning that the link between food and mood was examined at one point in time. The two were linked, but it isn't clear if poor moods led people to eat less-healthy food, or whether less-healthy food led people to experience poor moods. When other studies are examined, it appears likely that both effects occur—there is a potential for a feed-forward cycle between low mood, poor food choices, and a worsening mood.

Concerning the link between mood and food choices, it is clear that the ability to resist comforting snacks decreases with a negative mood. When in a bad mood, people seek immediate gratification (acting on the momentary impulse to make themselves feel better).[8] Food is part of this wish for immediate gratification. People want to feel better, and the next bag of chips offers some promise of distraction and relief. Interestingly, if people are led to believe that their mood will not change readily, then they don't tend to use such problematic strategies.[9]

There is also evidence that food selection has an impact on subsequent mood. In a large-scale study in Spain, for example, rates of depression in over 10,000 adults were examined over a more than 4-year period. In these people, 480 cases of new depression were documented, and a link between these new cases of depression and diet was evident. In general, greater adherence to a Mediterranean Diet (see below) was helpful for mood. Of specific foods, the consumption of more fruit and nuts was linked to lower rates of depression, and greater consumption of meats and whole-fat dairy products was linked to higher rates of depression. Similar supporting evidence comes from a large-scale study in England.[10] There, researchers examined the link between diet and depressed mood across 5 years in 3,486 adults. A high consumption of processed foods—characterized by processed meat, fried food, refined grains, high-fat dairy products, sweetened desserts, chocolates, and condiments—was linked to higher depression scores. On the other hand, a Mediterranean-type diet—in this case defined by fish, fruits, and vegetables—was linked to lower depression.

It is not clear what it is about these dietary patterns, and indeed whether it is the diet or some other associated factor, that influences depression. However, a Mediterranean diet tastes good, providing one striking reason for adopting it before all the mood evidence is in. In addition to good taste and good mood, there's another compelling reason to adopt a Mediterranean-type diet: physical health!

FOOD AND PHYSICAL HEALTH

Following a Mediterranean-type diet has clear health benefits. By diet, we mean what you eat, not how much you eat; we are not commenting on dieting in this book—lots of other books are available for that. The Mediterranean-type diet refers to the regular consumption of whole grains, nuts, fish, chicken, olive oil, and red wine (beer may be out, but wine is in). Considered together, an impressive amount of evidence shows that this pattern of eating is linked to reductions in overall death rates, rates of cardiovascular disease and deaths, rates of cancers and cancer-related deaths, and rates of neurodegenerative diseases like Alzheimer's disease or Parkinson's disease.[11] The exact characterization of the Mediterranean-type diet differs somewhat between studies, but our best summary of this diet is captured in Table 11.2. For reasons of good taste, good mood, and good health, we see no reason not to try to select meals using these items whenever possible. Use the following list to generate replacement meals and snacks for some of the processed foods, fried foods, meat, and high-fat dairy products in your diet.

EATING PATTERNS: GETTING THE MOST OUT OF EXERCISE

With regular exercise for mood, you have already taken a crucial step toward weight loss. With regular exercise, you are burning more calories while you exercise and building more muscles that can keep burning calories outside the exercise session. As you build more muscle with exercise, those muscles burn more calories, even when you are not working out. In addition, with a shift toward a Mediterranean-type diet, you will be eating foods that should maintain your pleasure in eating while offering you health and mood benefits. The next step for health is to make sure that you don't undo the weight loss benefits of exercise and the health promotion of the Mediterranean diet by eating more. As we discussed in Chapter 9, compensatory eating can undo some of your gains from exercise. The alternative is to focus on

Table 11.2. Guidelines for adopting a mediterranean diet

Increase foods from plant sources, preferably minimally processed:

- Get most of your food from plant sources, including fruits and vegetables, potatoes, breads and grains, beans, nuts, and seeds.
- Aim for 7–10 servings per day.
- Switch to whole-grain bread, cereals, and pastas, and brown rice.
- Choose a variety of minimally processed and seasonally fresh and locally grown foods, which maximizes their micronutrient and antioxidant content.

Increase consumption of nuts:

- Eat a handful of nuts daily, such as almonds, cashews, or walnuts.
- Avoid candied, honey-roasted, and heavily salted nuts.

Make olive oil your main source of fat:

- Use olive oil for your principal fat (or other oils rich in monounsaturated fats, such as canola or peanut oil) instead of butter, margarine, and other oils.
- Eat a high ratio of monounsaturated to saturated fat.

Choose fish and poultry over red meat:

- Eat fatty fish (such as mackerel, lake trout, herring, sardines, albacore tuna, and salmon) and poultry at least twice per week.
- Limit red meat consumption to a few times per month; when eaten, choose lean meat in small portions (size of a deck of cards).

Table 11.2. (Continued)

Eat a limited amount of low-fat dairy:

- Daily consumption of low to moderate amounts of cheese and yogurt.
- Choose low-fat and non-fat versions.

Make fruit your sweet snack of choice:

- Eat fresh fruit daily instead of high-sugar sweets.

Season food with spices:

- Use herbs and spices instead of salt to flavor meals.

Wine in moderation (optional):

- Consume moderate amounts of wine (about one to two glasses per day for men and one glass per day for women).
- Purple grape juice can be an alternative to wine.

---

a healthy diet, with no eating rewards on days of exercise. But, what should you do about hunger?

Hunger

Exercise will leave you feeling hungry. Exercise will also help you become better at not being pushed around by momentary feelings of hunger. In Chapter 8, we discussed mindfulness, the process of being aware of feelings of exertion in your body (feeling sweaty, breathless, and queasy) while not being overly influenced by these feelings. Just because you feel these sensations, you don't have to stop your run, bike, swim, etc. As we discussed in that chapter, mindfulness helps you to be aware of the range of events in your mind—sensations, feelings, thoughts—while not having to be too involved with any one of them. You choose what is best for you against a backdrop of both useful and less than useful thoughts or pleasant and unpleasant sensations. Apply this skill to temporary sensations of hunger and urges to snack.

Every urge to eat or every pang of hunger does not need to be met with eating. Indeed, discomfort with bodily sensations is linked to dysregulated eating. As you become comfortable with the range of bodily sensations that occur with exercise, transfer this ability to how you evaluate feelings in your gut ("Just as I became more comfortable with feelings of exertion, I can get comfortable with this subtle feeling in my stomach"). The key is deciding what the healthful level of eating is for your body, and then pursuing that level with a healthful choice of foods in line with a Mediterranean-type diet. If you are unsure of what you should eat (or if you have gotten feedback that you are under- or overeating), check with a nutritionist to get a sense of what your body requires for health. Once you set that level as a goal, enjoy your eating as much as possible, with diverse foods eaten across three or more healthy meals a day.

Thirst

Thirst deserves your attention. You do need to rehydrate your body after exercise. Do this with water. High-calorie drinks are an excellent way *to nullify* the calories burned during exercise. Even one large sweetened soda or sport drink can account for approximately 10% of daily recommended calories (check the label: some of these drinks are amazing sugar fests). More explicitly, we recommend an elimination of all ultra-sweetened drinks in favor of still or sparkling water. If you have been drinking sugary sodas, it will take you some time to find unsweetened sparkling water tasty, but it will happen with practice.

In successful change, people are creatures of *incrementalism*; changes that last often occur in a stepwise fashion. For example, giving up sweetened drinks can start with a shift from a sugared cola to a diet cola (first filing the cup 50/50 with diet cola, and then progressing to 100% diet soda across a week or two). But don't stop there. Also try to replace these drinks with pure water. This may take incremental action as well. Sparkling water with a twist of lime can be a fully satisfying drink on its own. But to be able to enjoy this drink, you need to lose the taste for super sweet. To work yourself to this point, try adding a sweetened juice to the sparkling water (cranberry juice cocktail, for example). Then, over time, reduce the juice content, watching your drink go from red to light pink as you use less and less juice and develop a greater taste for sparkling water alone. You don't have to pick sparkling water. We chose it as an example because we like it, and it nicely illustrates the incremental change that helps people change habits. And don't forget the tall glass, ice, and straw—it's often the little things that make a cold drink fun. Hydrate yourself well.

ARRANGING YOUR FOOD ENVIRONMENT

A clear theme of this book is how to arrange your environment so that you don't have to come up with your own motivation from deep within. We want you to put yourself in the position of having your environment motivate you. There is terrific evidence that this works well for healthy food choices.[12] Even subtle differences in effort appear to make a huge difference for food choices. For example, placing a bowl of candies one desk (6 feet) away, rather than on your desk, can lead to a 65% reduction in pieces of candy eaten.[13] In other words, use the choice architecture principles we reviewed in Chapter 4 to help yourself make healthy choices.

Excellent research shows that effort and serving ware can make a large difference in eating habits. First, don't make eating unhealthy food easy. Your efforts at promoting healthy eating start at the food store. If you don't buy high-fat foods, you can't eat them in a moment of weakness. Go to the food store after you have eaten, and when you are in a good mood, so that hunger and/or the desire for high-calorie comfort food cannot lead you astray. If you do have more unhealthy food at home, place these foods high up in the cabinet or pantry, and put the healthy food choices (e.g., fruits and nuts) within easy reach, such as in a bowl on the counter. And, when you serve food, consider the serving dish. For example, placing snack food in a single large bowl instead of two smaller bowls (same amount of food, just different bowls) leads people to serve themselves over 50% more. And once they serve themselves 50% more, they tend to eat this additional amount as well.[14]

This leads us to another consideration: People tend to load up their plate and eat what is on their plate. With larger plate sizes, people take and eat more food. If you want to eat less, then give yourself the free gift of calorie control that comes from having smaller plates. Smaller plates mean less consumption, and according to research, equal feelings of satiety.[15] We get used to eating and feeling full based on what is on the plate or in our bowls, so that, in many cases, we are more controlled by the *look* of a full plate than by the actual amount of calories. Oh, and the same goes for glassware. People perceive tall thin glasses as containing more liquid, which means that if you serve your guests in glassware that is short and wide, they will drink more liquid than they otherwise might.

These principles and what you can do to make them work for you are summarized in Table 11.3. The value of these strategies is that the effort does not have to come from you. By following these guidelines, you can use your environment to make healthful eating choices easier and more automatic.

Table 11.3. Altering one's personal environment to help reduce consumption

How environmental factors influence consumption	How one's personal environment can be altered to help reduce consumption
THE EATING ENVIRONMENT	
Eating atmospherics: Atmospherics influence eating duration	• Before completing a meal, have the breadbasket removed or have an entrée wrapped up "to go." The atmosphere of a long and relaxing dinner can then be enjoyed without the temptation to overeat. • Although soft music and candlelight can improve one's enjoyment of a meal, they have calorie intake consequences. Instead of lingering and eating dessert, enjoy a cup of coffee in the pleasant atmosphere.
Eating effort: Increased effort decreases consumption	• Store tempting foods in less-convenient locations (such as in a basement or in a top cupboard). • Do not leave serving bowls and platters on the dinner table. Keep second servings a safe distance away.

(Continued)

Table 11.3. (Continued)

How environmental factors influence consumption	How one's personal environment can be altered to help reduce consumption
Eating with others: Socializing influences meal duration and consumption norms.	• Decide on how much to eat prior to the meal, instead of during it. Order smaller quantities (e.g., half-sized portions) to avoid "keeping pace" during the meal. • Model the behavior of a person who appears to be eating the least or the most slowly.
Eating distractions: Distractions can initiate, obscure, and extend consumption	• Discourage "grazing" by focusing only on food. Try to eat only when sitting down, and do this at a distraction-free table. • Before eating a distracting meal or snack (such as eating while watching television or reading the newspaper), pre-serve the portions and allow no "refills."

THE FOOD ENVIRONMENT (THE FIVE S'S)

Salience of food: Salient food promotes salient hunger	• Eliminate the cookie jar, or replace it with a fruit bowl. • Wrap tempting foods in foil to make them less visible and more forgettable. • Place healthier, low-density foods in the front of the refrigerator and the less healthy foods in the back.

Table 11.3. (Continued)

How environmental factors influence consumption	How one's personal environment can be altered to help reduce consumption
Structure and variety of food assortments: Structure and perceived variety drives consumption.	• Avoid multiple bowls of the same food (such as at parties or receptions) because they increase perceptions of variety and stimulate consumption. • At buffets and receptions, avoid having more than two different foods on the plate at the same time. • To discourage others from overconsuming in a high-variety environment (such as at a reception or dinner party), arrange foods into organized patterns. Conversely, arrange foods into less-organized patterns to help stimulate consumption in the cafeterias of retirement homes and hospitals.
Size of food packages and portions: The size of packages and portions consumption norms.	• Repackage foods into smaller containers to suggest smaller consumption norms. • Plate smaller dinner portions in advance. • Never eat from a package. Always transfer food to a plate or bowl, to make portion estimation easier.

(Continued)

Table 11.3. (Continued)

How environmental factors influence consumption	How one's personal environment can be altered to help reduce consumption
Stockpiling of food: Stockpiled food is quickly consumed	• Out of sight is out of mind. Reduce the visibility of stockpiled foods by moving them to the basement or to a cupboard immediately after they are purchased. • Reduce the convenience of stockpiled foods by boxing them up or freezing them. • Stockpile healthy, low-energy-density foods to stimulate their consumption and to leave less room for their high-density counterparts.
Serving containers: Serving containers that are wide or large create consumption illusions	• Replace short, wide glasses with tall, narrow ones. • Reduce serving sizes and consumption by using smaller bowls and plates. • Use smaller spoons rather than larger ones when serving oneself or when eating from a bowl.

Figure from Wansink, B. (2004). Environmental factors that increase the food intake and consumption volume of unknowing consumers. *Annual Review of Nutrition, 24,* 471–472, reprinted with permission.

Considering these principles, take a walk through your home and look where your attention is directed. How does your home environment encourage you in terms of activity, eating, and sitting? If you thought seriously about your daily goals, and what sort of activities and eating habits you wanted to encourage, how would you change your rooms? What would be on display? Where would the television be? Then devote an hour or two to reorganizing a few key rooms to see if they can better support your goals. The following sections continue this theme: How can you take lessons learned from your exercise program and extend them for a more active and happier life?

HAVING AN ACTIVE LIFESTYLE

In this chapter, we have so far focused on some of the *trees*—providing information on ways to feed your body food that really sustains it, ways to use your body on a daily basis through movement that has protective effects over time, and ways to arrange your environment so that it supports your goals for healthy eating and moving. Now, it is time to view the *forest*. We believe that exercising for mood is the first step in a lifestyle transformation toward healthy activity. We want you to capitalize on the changing feelings of vitality in your body, so that you will act vitally on a daily basis. Examine your environment and your habits to see where you can increase your movement and your involvement. Below are eight small ways to start the transformation toward a fitter and happier you.

1. Stairs, Walking, and Play

Active vitality—that is our goal for your daily functioning. One practical aspect of active vitality is the adaptive use of your body on a daily and hourly basis. Here, we ask the question, "How can you feel your body and your muscles every day?" The use of stairs and walking provides the easiest solutions for most people. At home, is there a local store to which you can walk instead of drive? How about using the stairs at home or at work? When you stand to walk into another room, do you take a moment to stretch lightly or do a few leg lifts? Do you take a moment to do some light standing push-ups against the wall (where you place your feet 2 to 3 feet from the wall, your hands on the wall at shoulder level, lean in, then press yourself back out)? A few standing push-ups are not a workout (they last under 30 seconds), but they give you a chance to feel your muscles, to feel your vitality, and to be aware of your body as something that needs attention and care.

Part of the philosophy for helping yourself increase daily activity is to work against exercise and movement apathy. Walking, standing push-ups, and taking stairs all help keep you in a frame of mind of daily self-care and regular exercise. In fact, consider starting a daily routine of mini exercises—something light, on the order of daily sit-ups and push-ups. One way to do this is to schedule daily sit-ups and push-ups within 10 minutes of getting up. This is to become a habit, to happen every single day of your life. Pick a nice spot on your floor, and before your morning shower (and before you leave the bedroom), do the sit-ups and the push-ups. This could be as few as five of each (doing push-ups on your knees if needed). These are done to wake up your body and to remind you that taking care of your body is important. Your authors do this, and it is a terrific way to wake up, stretch out, and in the case of the sit-ups, avoid lower back pain.

Over time, increase the number of repetitions; we can testify that 40 sit-ups can provide as much back pain relief as three ibuprofen per day. And it is relatively easy to do a sit-ups or push-ups every

1 to 2 seconds. Think how brief this is: under 2 minutes for 30 sit-ups and 30 push-ups. We know you have time for that, no matter what your morning routine. And having done the routine, it means that you step into your shower, step outside your door, and step into your working life with a sense of being linked to your body and already being more . . . well, athletic.

Also, the goal of daily low-level exercise is that it makes it easier to move on to a full exercise session. That is, by having a daily moment of feeling your body and its movement early in the morning, it makes it so much more natural to have a fuller workout later in the day (or to use the daily sit-ups and push-ups as a warm-up for going out on a run, heading to the climbing wall, etc.). On the days on which you don't have a fuller workout, you still have the benefit of feeling your body and its movement.

And, do you play? Part of feeling vitality is in being able to use your body for more play. In Chapter 9, we provided you with a list of pleasant events. Many of those pleasant events can get easier and more joyful when you are in better shape. If you have children, think how you can both get more exercise and make use of your increasing fitness for better play. Instead of just listening to or watching the Nerf gun battle, be part of the Nerf gun battle. How well can you duck and crawl, bend and stretch, and dodge and run now that you have been exercising? On the beach and in the park, what does it feel like to be fully involved in a game of chase—to feel your heart pound from effort, as well as from the exhilaration of being part of the fun?

2. Team: Finding Your Community

Is there a team sport that would be fun? Would it be valuable at this point in your life to be part of a team? Social events are not just for fun: They appear to have a crucial link to health. In fact, one of the more surprising public health findings is the degree to which being part of a social group is linked to life. That's right: Being part of a group predicts a lower death rate. Specifically, having at least one social group activity a month, as compared to having none, is associated with a 50% reduction in death rate over the next year.[16] It is not exactly clear why this is the case. Being part of a group may be linked to other demographic, economic, and social factors, but even when some of these factors are accounted for, a link still exists between sociability and lower death rates.

It may be that being part of a larger group may provide an extra buffer against stress. Aside from all of the personal stress, family stress, or work stress that may assail us monthly, with occasional group activities, we experience a link to something larger and more independent from our own lives. It may provide a crucial change in focus from everyday issues. We don't know if this is the source of the effect, but we don't think you should wait to find out. Join a group. It's fun, it breaks up the weekly routine, it provides a larger frame of reference, and it links us with others. A monthly dancing lesson, a softball team, a reading club, a church group, a volunteer organization, or just regular dinner parties with friends—these are all important. And, in terms of furthering your vitality, do think about how a weekly or monthly group can further your movement and activity goals: Many yoga, dance, and exercise classes, and well as all the team sports, provide you with a way of getting more social contact while also gaining the benefits of exercise. See how you can spread your exercise involvement and the mood buffering effects of exercise by expanding your sense of team.

3. Resilience: Knowing What You Can Do

Exercise can be a powerful way of extending your sense of resilience in life. By *resilience*, we mean the ability to persist despite adversity.

We don't mean the ability to keep your head down and plow ahead despite the consequences. We would call this stoicism. Instead, we mean the ability to keep your head up, look around, and choose the best option, all despite the presence of adversity. This ability, as compared to head-down stoicism, can help you make good decisions in life.

Exercise has already given you good training for resilience. Throughout this book, we have described the process of awareness and persistence in exercise despite the feelings of exertion. The ability to start exercise even though you may not feel like it, and the ability to continue with exercise even though you have the urge to stop, helps build your ability to persist. In Chapter 8, we described this as the building of your effort muscle. We discussed saving up this muscle strength for when you really need it (using environment-driven motivation instead of the effort muscle whenever possible). We also discussed building strength in the effort muscle as you get better at persisting with exercise. In that same chapter, we also discussed mindfulness as a skill to help with persistence and to increase joy during exercise. Mindfulness is the "head-up" part of resilience. Mindfulness is the ability to consider all your needs, goals, and principles, despite the presence of distracting thoughts or feelings. Mindfulness is useful during exercise, and it is useful during moments of stress, to help you tolerate emotion while you choose the most useful response.

Marveling was introduced to you in Chapter 5, and involves having a curious interest in your emotional content. In terms of your self-coaching, it sounds like the following: "Hmmm, look how upset I am getting, I wonder why?" or "Wow, I really have an urge to get angry. Is that really going to serve me here?" Mindfully tolerating feelings of anger, for example, while you select a useful response is not much different from tolerating the feelings of breathlessness during exercise. The experiences share in common a devotion to your goals and the ability to tolerate internal sensations. This is a gift of exercise training, but it takes active application. Practice it.

4. Smiling: Approaching Life, Ready for Pleasure

In Chapter 8, we discussed the benefits of being aware of the expressions on your face, and in setting out a half smile on your face as part of pursuing more pleasure during exercise. Now, use the half smile as part of pursuing more pleasure in life. When you place a half smile on your face, it is as if you are orienting yourself toward finding the pleasurable aspects of the next few moments. And vigilance to the positive, rather than vigilance to the negative, has powerful effects on how stressful subsequent negative events feel, and how much they impact your emotions.[17] Being prepared to smile is a way of finding and embracing the good moments of your day.

Also, don't underestimate the power of a smile on your social world. It is striking the degree to which a smile can put others at ease. We recommend that you try the following. On a daily basis, try to greet at least five other people with eye contact and a smile. This number is to include those who you know well, as well as those you don't know. At least one target should be someone you don't know at all—say a clerk in a store. When getting your change, for example, don't just look at your hand, but look at the clerk's eyes, wait for her or him to meet your gaze, and then smile and say "Thank you." Do this expecting that it will be a positive experience for the clerk, and make sure to observe the clerk's eyes and facial expression for the impact of your smile. See what you get back. With just a brief smile, you may have changed how the day feels, for both of you.

5. Making Time

Exercise takes time. In Chapter 6, we had you think about whether you get this time back, with increased energy, clarity of thought, and vitality brought by the exercise itself. You also get the time back by staying alive longer due to the expected physical health benefits of exercise. More fun, more clarity, more life—it seems like a good investment of time. But, as we talk about extending the gains from exercise, for having a more active and involved life, we have to again face the question: How to find the time? One answer is to cut television and Internet time. Television time alone accounts for almost 20 hours each week for the average American (over half of total leisure time), and there's a proven link that the more time spent in front of the TV, the more likely you are to be overweight.[18]

Although there are a few extraordinary shows on television (your authors can testify to the pleasurable diversions brought by *Lost, Six Feet Under, Scrubs,* or *Rubicon*), it is a matter of keeping balance. Television watching is the pinnacle of passive activity: an ideal fit for when we are emotionally tired. Instead of reaching out to the world, the world comes to us. We do nothing; no demands and no effort. But how many hours per week do we really need such passive time? If you watch television for several hours a day, consider devoting just one of these hours to something else—social time, activity time, talking time. We only want you to do it if it brings you more joy. But to know if it brings you more joy, you will have to try it for several weeks. Look again at the Activity List provided in Chapter 9, and think about what you have not done for some time. If your life seems balanced and fun, make no changes. If not, take away an hour from television and see whether you get a better life in return. You don't have to know in advance what you are going to do with that daily hour; if nothing else, see what adventure you can find if you leave the hour open for new experiences.

6. Expanding Experiences

If you were to list the top ten memorable moments in your life, how many of them would be tied to major events in life, and how many to spontaneous moments? We want to make sure you keep this balance, to realize that many happy experiences are the products of small and spontaneous choices in life. But we are creatures of habit. We learn to get through life, and we continue to do those things that helped us get by, regardless of whether these things are still meaningful or the best option. But what if we push ourselves out of these habits and the self-imposed limitations of doing only what we know how to do?

As we discussed earlier, to really try something new, it helps to be open to being bad at it. To step away from personal perfectionism is almost always a step toward richer experiences. Trying out new sports and activities (say, "dance lessons", and most men will scatter to the edges of the room, or even better, run into another room) demands a willingness to struggle with something at the beginning. As you look to expand your activity goals, lower your guard and learn, not through your expectations ("I know what I like"), but through your experiences ("I was surprised by how much I liked...."). You will need time for such exploration (oh yeah, that is why we wrote #5 above), and you will need to remind yourself that you don't have to be good at something to enjoy it. In trying new things, notice what works for your life, independent of what you thought would work for your life.

7. Reflecting on Joy

Chapter 9 brought up the idea of *echoing*, of making sure that you reflect upon and relive moments of joy and well-being during the day. We asked you to do this with exercise (thinking back about the benefits and positive feelings felt during and after exercise), and we are now asking you to do this more generally. Specifically, practice giving extra attention to those moments when your life is working well. To do this, keep a record of these moments, using a well being *Diary*. We regularly ask patients in treatment to keep a well being Diary. We find that, no matter the level of anxiety or depression an individual is facing, he or she is able to find periods of relative well-being. These periods deserve focus. A well being Diary provides this focus. In the diary, you monitor the thoughts and events surrounding periods of well-being. Each evening, you are to record the time in the last 24 hours when you experienced the most well-being, describing what happened, what you thought, and how you felt.

The active recording of these moments of well-being has four purposes. First, it helps you become adept at not just remembering the problems of daily life, but in searching out the good moments. This is important, as good moments deserve your attention. Second, the diary helps you relive these moments. If anything deserves extra review in the evenings, it is what went well during the day. We want you to echo these good moments, to feel the pleasure again in the evening. Third, use this recording time to consider how to have similar moments again the next day. Fourth, over time, the diary provides you with valuable record of periods of enjoyment that can be reviewed and used for planning of future events.

8. Spreading Joy

Joy appears to be contagious. When researchers examine patterns of well-being in social networks, knowing happy people is a predictor of being happy yourself.[19] In fact, friends who become happy (and who live within a mile of one another) increase your probability of being happy by 25%. There is similar evidence for happiness effects from next-door neighbors. Spousal relationships are more complex, with evidence for less-direct effects, but still an 8% probability of happiness when he or she becomes happy. With the use of exercise to decrease your depression (depression appears to travel through social networks as well[20]) and increase your well-being, we hope to see an increase in happiness in those who care about you. Your happiness serves your network, and it ultimately serves us. Your smiles, mindfulness, resilience, happiness, and fitness eventually have a chance to go through your social network, to friends of friends, to our friends, and to us. So, for our sake and yours, be happy and spread joy.

Resources

Here, you will find a number of resources to help with the maintenance of your exercise program and to aid in the treatment of depression and anxiety and improve well-being. For exercise and mood logs, as well as for calculators and other information related to the book, we direct you to http://www.exercise4mood.com. Other resources are categorized below by common questions we have received over the years.

1. Where Can I Learn More About The Nature And Treatment Of Depression And Anxiety?

National Institute of Mental Health (NIMH)
6001 Executive Boulevard Room 8184, MSC 9663
Bethesda, MD 20892-9663
Telephone: 301-443-4513
Fax: 301-443-4279
E-mail: nimhinfo@nih.gov
Website: http://www.nimh.nih.gov

The NIMH is a division of the National Institutes of Health (NIH) devoted to mental health. The NIMH aims to diminish the burden of mental illness through research.

The International Foundation for Research and Education on Depression (iFred)
PO Box 17598
Baltimore, MD 21297-1598
Fax: 443-782-0739
E-mail: info@ifred.org
Website: http://www.ifred.org/

iFred is an organization dedicated to helping research the causes of depression, to support those dealing with depression, and to combat the stigma associated with depression.

Anxiety Disorders Association of America (ADAA)

8730 Georgia Avenue
Silver Spring, MD 20910
Telephone: 240-485-1001
Fax: 240-485-1035
Website: http:/www.adaa.org

The mission of the ADAA is to promote the prevention, treatment, and cure of anxiety and stress-related disorders through advocacy, education, training, and research.

National Alliance for the Mentally Ill (NAMI)

200 North Glebe Road, Suite 1015
Arlington, VA 22203-3754
Telephone: 703-524-7600
Website: http://www.nami.org

The NAMI is a support and advocacy organization of consumers, families, and friends of people with severe mental illness and has more than 1,200 state and local affiliates. Local affiliates often give guidance to finding treatment.

National Mental Health Association (NMHA)

1021 Prince Street
Alexandria, VA 22314-2971
Telephone: 703-684-7722; 1-800-969-6642
Fax: 703-684-5968
Website: http://www.nmha.org

The NMHA is an association that works with 340 affiliates to promote mental health through advocacy, education, research, and services.

American Psychiatric Association (APA)

1400 K Street N.W.
Washington, DC 20005
Telephone: 888-357-7924
Fax: 202-682-6850
E-mail: apa@psych.org
Website: http://www.psych.org/

The American Psychiatric Association is a medical society of physicians specializing in the diagnosis and treatment of mental and emotional illnesses and substance use disorders.

American Psychological Association (APA)
750 First Street N.E.
Washington, DC 20002
Phone: 202-336-5500
Website: http://www.apa.org/

The APA is the largest scientific and professional organization representing psychology in the United States. It seeks to advance psychology as a science, a profession, and a means of promoting human welfare.

Association for Behavioral and Cognitive Therapies (ABCT)
305 7th Avenue, 16th Floor
New York, NY 10001
Telephone: 212-647-1890
Fax: 212-647-1865
Website: http://www.abct.org

The ABCT is an interdisciplinary organization committed to the advancement of a scientific approach to the understanding and amelioration of problems of the human condition. These aims are achieved through the investigation and application of behavioral, cognitive, and other evidence-based principles to assessment, prevention, and treatment.

2. Where Can I Find A Therapist?

We recommend visiting the "find a therapist" websites of the following organizations:

Anxiety Disorders Association of America
http://www.adaa.org/findatherapist

Association for Behavioral and Cognitive Therapies
http://www.abct.org/Members/?m=FindTherapist&fa=FT_Form&nolm=1

Academy of Cognitive Therapy
http://www.academyofct.org/Library/CertifiedMembers/Index.asp?FolderID=1137

American Psychological Association
http://locator.apa.org/

3. Where Can I Find The Public Health Recommendations For Exercise?

The physical activity guidelines for Americans were published in 2008 and can be found on the U.S. Department of Health and Human Services website at http://www.health.gov/paguidelines/

Other related information is made available by:

The American College of Sports Medicine
401 West Michigan Street
Indianapolis, IN 46202-3233
Telephone: 317-637-9200
Fax: 317-634-7817
Website: http://www.acsm.org/

The American College of Sports Medicine promotes and integrates scientific research, education, and practical applications of sports medicine and exercise science to maintain and enhance physical performance, fitness, health, and quality of life.

4. What Are Some Websites That Can Help Me As I Try To Establish An Exercise Routine?

Below is a selection of websites that the authors have found to be helpful for their own exercise, as well as in assisting their patients.

1. http://www.mapmyrun.com

Mapymyrun.com allows you to log on and find a local path to walk, run, bicycle, etc. It also includes information such as distances, maps, and other's reviews, ratings, and commentary of the path as well as other exercise events in the area. *Requires log in.

2. http://www.dietdoctor.com

Dietdoctor.com gives you information on exercise, diet myths, and health, as well as on a wide array of links and information on different diet regimes. The main focus of this website is in fact on diets and the truth about which ones work and don't work, although it includes links to exercise and workout programs as well.

3. http://www.fitclick.com

Fitclick.com provides a forum to discuss diet and exercise strategies and issues. Although it is set up similar to a social network site (i.e., Facebook) with a profile page, friends, etc., it is essentially a support system that provides useful links and a personalized fitness plan. *Requires log in.

4. http://www.exercise.com

Exercise.com provides links to exercise, equipment, diet and nutrition, and news and research articles. It even includes a local section where you can look up events in your area that you can join. It is similar to fitclick.com, but provides more links and resources than fitting to your personal needs through a profile page. *Requires log in.

5. http://www.webmd.com/fitness-exercise/default.htm

The Health and Fitness section of WebMD provides a vast array of articles both from research and the medical field along with individual reviews and commentary. It also offers thousands of valuable facts, links, and free connections to experts from accredited sources in the medical and health fields.

6. http://www.nhesa.org

Nhesa.org is the National Health & Exercise Science Association website that promotes healthy lifestyle choices, as well as research and insights into diet and exercise. This also provides connections to other national health associations events that are free to attend. *Requires log in.

7. http://www.fitness.gov

Fitness.gov is the President's Council on Fitness, Sports, & Nutrition main webpage that connects you to other resources for fitness. Along with advertising for its own cause, it lists links for other resources through the government for fitness, sports, nutrition, and general health, such as "Fitness Fundamentals: Guidelines for Personal Exercise Programs" and "United We Serve/Let's Read. Let's Move. Initiative."

8. http://www.crossfit.com

Crossfit is a "program [that] delivers a fitness that is, by design, broad, general, and inclusive" yet is "designed for universal scalability making it the perfect application for any committed individual regardless of experience." Besides being a worldwide program, you are able to train on your own with their instructions online, or find a group in a city near you and join the group for a fee.

9. http://www.campgladiator.com

Camp Gladiator is found mainly in Texas and Oklahoma, but quickly spreading. It provides group training as well as games. Although you have to pay to join, it is a fun group alternative to the usual gym scene.

10. http://www.usafit.com/

In the USA FIT program, participants challenge themselves, through running or walking, in small but ever-increasing doses. Then, after 6 months, many take and pass the final trial: 26.2 miles of a marathon. And you know what? Almost anyone can do it.

5. How Can I Learn More About Sport Promotion In Children?

1. http://www.worldfit.org/

World Fit is an initiative of the US Olympians Association. It is a walking program for middle school students, with the mission of curbing childhood obesity and improving overall health and attitudes toward fitness.

2. http://www.womenssportsfoundation.org

Women's Sports Foundation has the mission of advancing the lives of girls and women through sport and physical activity. The program was founded by Billie Jean King in 1974. The website provides a wealth of information for athletes, parents, coaches, schools, and other organizations.

6. Where Can I Learn About Exercise And Major Medical Conditions?

Exercise is often recommended as a strategy to aid both the mood challenges and risk factors associated with major medical illnesses such as cancer, heart disease, and diabetes. However, finding the appropriate stage for and level of exercise may be challenging. In addition to direct consultation with your physician, the following websites may provide valuable information on exercise in the context of illness recovery.

American Diabetes Association
http://www.diabetes.org/

Diabetes Society
www.diabetessociety.org

Juvenile Diabetes Research Foundation International
http://www.jdrf.org/

American Cancer Society
http://www.cancer.org/

Lance Armstrong Foundation
http://www.livestrong.org/

Susan G. Komen for the Cure
http://ww5.komen.org/

The Leukemia & Lymphoma Society
www.leukemia-lymphoma.org

Lung Cancer Foundation of America
www.lcfamerica.org

National Childhood Cancer Foundation
www.curesearch.org

American Heart Association
www.heart.org

Women's Heart Foundation
www.womensheart.org

7. What Are Some Tools For Tracking My Progress?

For logging your exercise, as well as for logging your mood changes, the following forms can be of value.

1. Exercise Planning
2. Exercise for Mood Log
3. Quick Inventory of Depressive Symptomatology
4. Exercise Practice Log for Panic-related Concerns

Resources Log 1. My exercise schedule

Month:

Sunday	Monday	Tuesday	Wednesday	Thursday	Friday	Saturday

Resources Log 2. Exercise for mood log

This log is to help me keep track of my exercise goals for mood by focusing on the importance of exercise several days a week.

Week Number _____

	Day 1 Date: __/__	Day 2 Date: __/__	Day 3 Date: __/__	Day 4 Date: __/__	Day 5 Date: __/__	Day 6 Date: __/__	Day 7 Date: __/__
Day of the week							
Exercise completed ($\checkmark$)							
Time of day of exercise							
Type of exercise completed							
Intensity (% HR_{max})							
Duration (minutes)							
Pre-exercise Feelings/Mood							
Post-exercise Feelings/Mood							

Resources Log 3. The QIDS

The Quick Inventory of Depressive Symptomatology (16-Item) (Self-Report) (QIDS-SR16)

Name or ID: _____   Date: _____

CHECK THE ONE RESPONSE TO EACH ITEM THAT BEST DESCRIBES YOU FOR THE PAST SEVEN DAYS.

During the past seven days...

1. Falling Asleep:

☐ 0 I never take longer than 30 minutes to fall asleep.

☐ 1 I take at least 30 minutes to fall asleep, less than half the time.

☐ 2 I take at least 30 minutes to fall asleep, more than half the time.

☐ 3 I take more than 60 minutes to fall asleep, more than half the time.

2. Sleep During the Night

☐ 0 I do not wake up at night.

☐ 1 I have a restless, light sleep with a few brief awakenings each night.

☐ 2 I wake up at least once a night, but I go back to sleep easily.

☐ 3 I awaken more than once a night and stay awake for 20 minutes or more, more than half the time.

3. Waking Up Too Early:

☐ 0 Most of the time, I awaken no more than 30 minutes before I need to get up.

☐ 1 More than half the time, I awaken more than 30 minutes before I need to get up.

☐ 2 I almost always awaken at least one hour or so before I need to, but I go back to sleep eventually.

☐ 3 I awaken at least one hour before I need to, and can't go back to sleep.

4. Sleeping Too Much:

☐ 0 I sleep no longer than 7-8 hours/night, without napping during the day.

☐ 1 I sleep no longer than 10 hours in a 24-hour period including naps.

☐ 2 I sleep no longer than 12 hours in a 24-hour period including naps.

☐ 3 I sleep longer than 12 hours in a 24-hour period including naps.

Enter the highest score on any 1 of the 4 sleep items (1–4 above) _____

During the past seven days...

5. Feeling Sad:

☐ 0 I do not feel sad.

☐ 1 I feel sad less than half the time.

☐ 2 I feel sad more than half the time.

☐ 3 I feel sad nearly all of the time.

Please complete either 6 or 7   (not both)

6. Decreased Appetite:

☐ 0 There is no change in my usual appetite.

☐ 1 I eat somewhat less often or lesser amounts of food than usual.

☐ 2 I eat much less than usual and only with personal effort.

☐ 3 I rarely eat within a 24-hour period, and only with extreme personal effort or when others persuade me to eat.

- OR -

7. Increased Appetite:

☐ 0 There is no change from my usual appetite.

☐ 1 I feel a need to eat more frequently than usual.

☐ 2 I regularly eat more often and/or greater amounts of food than usual.

☐ 3 I feel driven to overeat both at mealtime and between meals.

Please complete either 8 or 9   (not both)

8. Decreased Weight (Within the Last Two Weeks):

☐ 0 I have not had a change in my weight.

☐ 1 I feel as if I have had a slight weight loss.

☐ 2 I have lost 2 pounds or more.

☐ 3 I have lost 5 pounds or more.

- OR -

9. Increased Weight (Within the Last Two Weeks):

☐ 0 I have not had a change in my weight.

☐ 1 I feel as if I have had a slight weight gain.

☐ 2 I have gained 2 pounds or more.

☐ 3 I have gained 5 pounds or more.

Enter the highest score on any 1 of the 4 appetite/weight change items (6–9 above) _____

Scoring: The total score for the QIDS is the sum of the following: the highest score of items 1-4, item 5, the highest score of items 6-9, item 10, item 11, item 12, item 13, item 14, and the highest score of items 15 and 16. Total scores range between 0 and 27, with higher scores indicating greater symptoms of depression. Track these scores over time. Total Score for this week _____.

The Quick Inventory of Depressive Symptomatology (16-Item) (Self-Report) (QIDS-SR$_{16}$)

During the past seven days...

10. Concentration / Decision Making:

☐ 0   There is no change in my usual capacity to concentrate or make decisions.

☐ 1   I occasionally feel indecisive or find that my attention wanders.

☐ 2   Most of the time, I struggle to focus my attention or to make decisions.

☐ 3   I cannot concentrate well enough to read or cannot make even minor decisions.

11. View of Myself:

☐ 0   I see myself as equally worthwhile and deserving as other people.

☐ 1   I am more self-blaming than usual.

☐ 2   I largely believe that I cause problems for others.

☐ 3   I think almost constantly about major and minor defects in myself.

12. Thoughts of Death or Suicide:

☐ 0   I do not think of suicide or death.

☐ 1   I feel that life is empty or wonder if it's worth living.

☐ 2   I think of suicide or death several times a week for several minutes.

☐ 3   I think of suicide or death several times a day in some detail, or I have made specific plans for suicide or have actually tried to take my life.

13. General Interest

☐ 0   There is no change from usual in how interested I am in other people or activities.

☐ 1   I notice that I am less interested in people or activities.

☐ 2   I find I have interest in only one or two of my formerly pursued activities.

☐ 3   I have virtually no interest in formerly pursued activities.

During the past seven days...

14. Energy Level:

☐ 0   There is no change in my usual level of energy.

☐ 1   I get tired more easily than usual.

☐ 2   I have to make a big effort to start or finish my usual daily activities (for example, shopping, homework, cooking, or going to work).

☐ 3   I really cannot carry out most of my usual daily activities because I just don't have the energy.

15. Feeling Slowed Down:

☐ 0   I think, speak, and move at my usual rate of speed.

☐ 1   I find that my thinking is slowed down or my voice sounds dull or flat.

☐ 2   It takes me several seconds to respond to most questions and I'm sure my thinking is slowed.

☐ 3   I am often unable to respond to questions without extreme effort.

16. Feeling Restless:

☐ 0   I do not feel restless.

☐ 1   I'm often fidgety, wringing my hands, or need to shift how I am sitting.

☐ 2   I have impulses to move about and am quite restless.

☐ 3   At times, I am unable to stay seated and need to pace around.

Enter the highest score on either of the 2 psychomotor items (15 or 16 above) _____

Resources Log 4. Exercise practice log for panic-related concerns

Date of Exercise:_____

What sensations did you experience during your exercise?

_____

_____

How intense were the sensations during your workout (0—100)?

Beginning :

Half-way :

Toward the end :

What was your anxiety level throughout the session (0–100)?

Beginning :

Half-way :

Toward the end :

What were the actual consequences of the sensations that you experienced, particularly when you tried a mindful perspective on these sensations?

_____

_____

How did these consequences differ from any specific fears you had about these sensations, or urges you had to control the sensations?

_____

_____

What do you want to tell yourself about these sensations now?

_____

_____

_____

Physical Activity Readiness Questionnaire (PAR-Q)

If you are between the ages of 15 and 69, the PAR-Q will tell you if you should check with your doctor before engaging in physical activity. Common sense is your best guide when you answer these questions. Please read them carefully and answer each one honestly by checking Yes or No.

Yes	No	
☐	☐	1. Has your doctor ever said that you have a heart condition and that you should only do physical activity recommended by a doctor?
☐	☐	2. Do you feel pain in your chest when you do physical activity?
☐	☐	3. In the past month, have you had chest pain when you were not doing physical activity?
☐	☐	4. Do you lose your balance because of dizziness, or do you ever lose consciousness?
☐	☐	5. Do you have a bone or joint problem (e.g., back, knee, or hip) that could be made worse by a change in your physical activity?
☐	☐	6. Is your doctor currently prescribing drugs (e.g., water pills) for high blood pressure or a heart condition?
☐	☐	7. Do you know of any other reason why you should not engage in physical activity?

If you answered Yes to one or more questions, talk to your doctor **before** beginning a physical activity program.

If you answered No to all questions, you can be reasonably sure that you can start becoming more physically active.

REFERENCES

Chapter 2

1. Stephens, T. (1988). Physical activity and mental health in the United States and Canada: Evidence from four popular surveys. *Preventive Medicine, 17,* 35–47.
2. Hassmen, P., Koivula, N., & Uutela, A. (2000). Physical exercise and psychological well-being: A population study in Finland. *Preventive Medicine, 30,* 17–25.
3. Goodwin, R. D. (2003). Association between physical activity and mental disorders among adults in the United States. *Preventive Medicine, 36,* 698–703.
4a. Kessler, R. C., Berglund, P., Demler, O., Jin, R., Merikangas, K. R., & Walters, E. E. (2005). Lifetime prevalence and age-of-onset distributions of DSM-IV disorders in the national comorbidity survey replication. *Archives of General Psychiatry, 62,* 593–602.
4b. Farmer, M. E., Locke, B. Z., Mosciki, E. K., Dannenberg, A. L., Larson, D. B., & Radloff, L. S. (1998). Physical activity and depressive symptoms: The NHANES I Epidemiologic Follow-up Study. *American Journal of Epidemiology, 128,* 1340–1351.
4c. Camacho, T. C., Roberts, R. E., Lazarus, N. B., Kaplan, G. A., & Cohen, R. D. (1991). Physical activity and depression: Evidence from the Alameda County Study. *American Journal of Epidemiology, 134,* 220–231.
4d. Paffenbarger, R. S., Jr., Lee, I. M., & Leung, R. (1994). Physical activity and personal characteristics associated with depression and suicide in American college men. *Acta Psychiatrica Scandanavia, 89*(Suppl. 377), 16–22.

5. Paffenbarger, R. S., Jr., Lee, I. M., & Leung, R. (1994). Physical activity and personal characteristics associated with depression and suicide in American college men. *Acta Psychiatrica Scandanavia, 89*(Suppl. 377), 16–22.

6. Strohle, A., Hofler, M., Pfister, H., Muller, A. G., Hoyer, J., Wittchen, H. U., & Lieb, R. (2007). Physical activity and prevalence and incidence of mental disorders in adolescents and young adults. *Psychological Medicine, 37,* 1657–1666.

7. Conn, V. S. (2010). Depressive symptom outcomes of physical activity interventions: Meta-analysis findings. *Annals of Behavioral Medicine, 39,* 128–138.

8. Eaton, W. W., Shao, H., Nestadt, G., Lee, H. B., Bienvenu, O. J., & Zandi, P. (2008). Population-based study of first onset and chronicity in major depressive disorder. *Archives of General Psychiatry, 65,* 513–520.

9. Kessler, R. C., Berglund, P., Demler, O., Jin, R., Merikangas, K. R., & Walters, E. E. (2005). Lifetime prevalence and age-of-onset distributions of DSM-IV disorders in the national comorbidity survey replication. *Archives of General Psychiatry, 62,* 593–602.

10. Bruce, S. E., Yonkers, K. A., Otto, M. W., Eisen, J. L., Weisberg, R. B., Pagano, M., et al. (2005). Influence of psychiatric comorbidity on recovery and recurrence in generalized anxiety disorder, social phobia, and panic disorder: A 12-year prospective study. *American Journal of Psychiatry, 162,* 1179–1187.

11. Sothmann, M. S., Buckworth, J., Claytor, R. P., Cox, R. H., White-Welkley, J. E., & Dishman, R. K. (1996). Exercise training and the cross-stressor adaptation hypothesis. *Exercise and Sport Sciences Reviews, 24,* 267–287.

12a. Throne, L. C., Bartholomew, J. B., Craig, J., & Farrar, R. P. (2000). Stress reactivity in fire fighters: An exercise intervention. *International Journal of Stress Management, 7,* 235–246.

12b. Sothmann, M. S., Buckworth, J., Claytor, R. P., Cox, R. H., White-Welkley, J. E., & Dishman, R. K. (1996). Exercise training and the cross-stressor adaptation hypothesis. *Exercise and Sport Sciences Reviews, 24,* 267–287.

13a. Hammen, C. (2005). Stress and depression. *Annual Review of Clinical Psychology, 1,* 293–319.

13b. Heim, C., & Nemeroff, C. B. (1999). The impact of early adverse experiences on brain systems involved in the pathophysiology of anxiety and affective disorders. *Biological Psychiatry, 46,* 1509–1522.

14. Mazure, C. M. (1998). Life stressors as risk factors in depression. *Clinical Psychology: Science & Practice, 5,* 291–313.

15a. Coppen, A. (1967). The biochemistry of affective disorders. *British Journal of Psychiatry, 113,* 1237–1264.

15b. Meltzer, H. (1989). Serotonergic dysfunction in depression. *British Journal of Psychiatry (Supplement), 8,* 25–31.

16. Goodnick, P. J., & Goldstein, B. J. (1998). Selective serotonin reuptake inhibitors in affective disorders-II. Efficacy and quality of life. *Journal of Psychopharmacology, 12*, 21–54.

17a. Dey, S., Singh, R. H., & Dey, P. K. (1992). Exercise training: Significance of regional alterations in serotonin metabolism of rat brain in relation to antidepressant effect of exercise. *Physiology and Behavior, 52*, 1095–1099.

17b. Wilson, W., & Marsden, C. (1996). In vivo measurement of extracellular serotonin in the ventral hippocampus during treadmill running. *Behavioural Pharmacology, 7*, 101–104.

17c. Meeusen, R., Thorré, K., Chaouloff, F., Sarre, S., De Meirleir, K., Ebinger, G., et al. (1996). Effects of tryptophan and/or acute running on extracellular 5-HT and 5-HIAA levels in the hippocampus of food-deprived rats. *Brain Research, 740*, 245–252.

18. Wilson, W., & Marsden, C. (1996). In vivo measurement of extracellular serotonin in the ventral hippocampus during treadmill running. *Behavioural Pharmacology, 7*, 101–104.

19a. Meeusen, R., & De Meirleir, K. (1995). Exercise and brain neurotransmission. *Sports Medicine, 20*, 160–188.

19b. Dunn, A. L., & Dishman, R. K. (1991). Exercise and the neurobiology of depression. *Exercise and Sport Sciences Reviews, 19*, 41–98.

20. Broocks, A., Schweiger, U., & Pirke, K. M. (1991). The influence of semistarvation-induced hyperactivity on hypothalamic serotonin metabolism. *Physiology & Behavior, 50*, 385–388.

21a. Broocks, A., Meyer, T., George, A., Hillmer-Vogel, U., Meyer, D., Bandelow, B., et al. (1999). Decreased neuroendocrine responses to meta-chlorophenylpiperazine (m-CPP) but normal responses to ipsapirone in marathon runners. *Neuropsychopharmacology, 20*, 150–161.

21b. Broocks, A., Meyer, T., Gleiter, C. H., Hillmer-Vogel, U., George, A., Bartmann, U., & Bandelow, B. (2001). Effect of aerobic exercise on behavioral and neuroendocrine responses to meta-chlorophenylpiperazine and to ipsapirone in untrained healthy subjects. *Psychopharmacology (Berl), 155*, 234–141.

21c. Broocks, A., Meyer, T., Opitz, M., Bartmann, U., Hillmer-Vogel, U., George, A., et al. (2003). 5-HT1A responsivity in patients with panic disorder before and after treatment with aerobic exercise, clomipramine or placebo. *European Neuropsychopharmacology, 13*, 153–164.

22. Blumenthal, J. A., Babyak, M. A., Doraiswamy, M., Watkins, L., Hoffman, B. M., Barbour, K. A., et al. (2007). Exercise and pharmacotherapy in the treatment of major depressive disorder. *Psychosomatic Medicine, 69*, 587–596.

23a. Hopko, D. R., Lejuez, C. W., Ruggiero, K. J., & Eifert, G. H. (2003). Contemporary behavioral activation treatments for depression: Procedures principles and progress. *Clinical Psychology Review, 23*, 699–717.

23b. Jacobson, N. S., Martell, C. R., & Dimidjian, S. (2001). Behavioral activation treatment for depression: Returning to contextual roots. *Clinical Psychology: Science and Practice, 8,* 255–270.

24a. Broman-Fulks, J. J., Berman, M. E., Rabian, B., & Webster, M. J. (2004). Effects of aerobic exercise on anxiety sensitivity. *Behaviour Research and Therapy, 42,* 125–136.

24b. Broman-Fulks, J. J., & Storey, K. M. (2008). Evaluation of a brief aerobic exercise intervention for high anxiety sensitivity. *Anxiety, Stress & Coping: An International Journal, 21,* 117–128.

24c. Smits, J. A., Berry, A. C., Rosenfield, D., Powers, M. B., Behar, E., & Otto, M. W. (2008). Reducing anxiety sensitivity with exercise. *Depression & Anxiety, 25,* 689–699.

25. Reiss, S., Peterson, R. P., Gursky, D. M., & McNally, R. J. (1986). Anxiety sensitivity, anxiety frequency, and the prediction of fearfulness. *Behaviour Research and Therapy, 24,* 1–8.

26a. Cox, B. J., Enns, M. W., Freeman, P., & Walker, J. R. (2001). Anxiety sensitivity and major depression: Examination of affective state dependence. *Behaviour Research and Therapy, 39,* 1349–1356.

26b. Schmidt, N. B., Zvolensky, M. Z., & Maner, J. K. (2006). Anxiety sensitivity: Prospective prediction of panic attacks and Axis I pathology. *Journal of Psychiatric Research, 40,* 691–699.

26c. Taylor, S., Koch, W. J., & McNally, R. J. (1992). How does anxiety sensitivity vary across the anxiety disorders? *Journal of Anxiety Disorders, 6,* 249–259.

27. Stathopoulou, G., Powers, M. B., Berry, A. C., Smits, J. A. J., & Otto, M. W. (2006). Exercise interventions for mental health: A quantitative and qualitative review. *Clinical Psychology: Science & Practice, 13,* 179–193.

28a. Ossip-Klein, D. J., Bowman, E. D., Osborn, K. M., McDougall-Willson, I. B., & Neimeyer, R. A. (1987). Running versus weight-lifting in the treatment of depression. *Journal of Consulting and Clinical Psychology, 55,* 748–754.

28b. Martinsen, E. W., Hoffart, A., & Solberg, O. (1989). Comparing aerobic with nonaerobic forms of exercise in the treatment of clinical depression: A randomized trial. *Comprehensive Psychiatry, 30,* 324–331.

29. Dunn, A. L., Trivedi, M. H., Kampert, J. B., Clark, C. G., & Chambliss, H. O. (2005). Exercise treatment for depression: Efficacy and dose response. *American Journal of Preventive Medicine, 28,* 1–8.

30. Ekkekakis, P. (2003). Pleasure and displeasure from the body: Perspectives from exercise. *Cognition and Emotion, 17*(2), 213–239.

31a. Long, B. C., & van Stavel, R. (1995). Effects of exercise training on anxiety: A meta-analysis. *Journal of Applied Sport Psychology, 7,* 167–189.

31b. Petruzzello, S. J., Landers, D. M., Hatfield, B. D., Kubitz, K. A., & Salazar, W. (1991). A meta-analysis on the anxiety-reducing effects of acute and chronic exercise. Outcomes and mechanisms. *Sports Medicine, 11,* 143–182.

Chapter 3

1a. Lee, I. M., & Paffenbarger, R. S. (2001). Do physical activity and physical fitness avert premature mortality? *Exercise and Sport Science Reviews, 24,* 135–171.

1b. Lee, I. M., Hsieh, C. C., & Paffenbarger, R. S. (1995). Exercise intensity and longevity in men. The Harvard alumni health study. *Journal of the American Medical Association, 274,* 1132–1133.

1c. Haennel, R. G., & Lemire, F. (2002). Physical activity to prevent cardiovascular disease. How much is enough? *Canadian Family Physician, 48,* 65–71.

1d. Berlin, J. A., & Colditz, G. A. (1990). A meta-analysis of physical activity in the prevention of coronary heart disease. *American Journal of Epidemiology, 134,* 232–234.

2. Your government is working for you. For examples of public initiatives for reducing risk factors for death among Americans see http://www.cancer.gov/, http://www2.niddk.nih.gov/, and http://www.cdc.gov/Features/HaltingObesity/

3. CDC. (n.d.) *Physical activity statistics.* Retrieved fromhttp://www.cdc.gov/nccdphp/dnpa/physical/stats/leisure_time.htm

4. Oettingen, G., & Mayer, D. (2002). The motivating function of thinking about the future: Expectations versus fantasies. *Journal of Personality and Social Psychology, 83,* 1198–1212.

5. Madden, G. J., & Bickel, W. K. (2010). *Impulsivity: The behavioral and neurological science of discounting.* Washington, DC: American Psychological Association.

6. Vital signs: Current cigarette smoking among adults aged > or =18 years—United States, 2009. (2010). *MMWR: Morbidity and Mortality Weekly Report, 59,* 1135–1140.

7a. Carver, C. S., & Scheier, M. F. (2008). Feedback processes in the simultaneous regulation of action and affect. In J. Y. Shah, & W. L. Gardner (Eds.), *Handbook of Motivational Science* (pp. 308–324). New York: Guilford.

7b. Tice, D. M., Batslavsky, E., & Baumeiser, R. F. (2001). Emotional distress regulation takes precedence over impulse control. If you feel bad, do it! *Journal of Personality and Social Psychology, 8,* 53–67.

8. Ekkekakis, P. (2003). Pleasure and displeasure from the body: Perspectives from exercise. *Cognition and Emotion, 17,* 213–239.

9. Ekkekakis, P. (2003). Pleasure and displeasure from the body: Perspectives from exercise. *Cognition and Emotion, 17,* 213–239.

10. Williams, D. M., Dunsiger, S., Ciccolo, J. T., Lewis, B. A., Albrecht, A. E., & Marcus, B. H. (2008). Acute affective response to a moderate-intensity exercise stimulus predicts physical activity participation 6 and 12 months later. *Psychology of Sport and Exercise, 9,* 231–245.

11a. Acevedo, E. O., Rinehardt, K. F., & Kraemer, R. R. (1994). Perceived exertion and affect at varying intensities of running. *Research Quarterly for Exercise and Sport, 65,* 372–376.

11b. Hardy, C. J., & Rejeski, W. J. (1989). Not what, but how one feels: The measurement of affect during exercise. *Journal of Sport & Exercise Psychology, 11*, 304–317.

12a. Ekkekakis, P., Hall, E. E., & Petruzzello, S. J. (1999). Cognitive and physiological correlates of affect during a maximal exercise test. *Journal of Sport & Exercise Psychology, 21*, S40.

12b. Ekkekakis, P., & Petruzzello, S. J. (2002). Analysis of the affect measurement conundrum in exercise psychology: IV. A conceptual case for the affect circumplex. *Psychology of Sport & Exercise, 3*, 35–63.

13. Hart, E. A., Leary, M. R., & Rejeski, W. J. (1989). The measurement of social physique anxiety. *Journal of Sport & Exercise Psychology, 11*, 94–104.

14a. Focht, B. C., & Hausenblas, H. A. (2003). State anxiety responses to acute exercise in women with high social physique anxiety. *Journal of Sport and Exercise Psychology, 25*, 123–144.

14b. Focht, B. C., & Hausenblas, H. A. (2004). Perceived evaluative threat and state anxiety during exercise in women with social physique anxiety. *Journal of Applied Sport Psychology, 16*, 361–368.

14c. Katula, J. A., McAuley, E., Mihalko, S. L., & Bane, S. M. (1998). Mirror, mirror on the wall … Exercise environment influences on self-efficacy. *Journal of Social Behavior and Personality, 13*, 319–332.

14d. Martin-Ginis, K. A., Jung, M. E., & Gauvin, L. (2003). To see or not to see: Effects of exercising in mirrored environments on sedentary women's feeling states and self-efficacy. *Health Psychology, 22*, 354–361.

15. Smits, J. A. J., Tart, C. D., Presnell, K., Rosenfield, D., & Otto, M. W. (2010). Identifying potential barriers to physical activity adherence: Anxiety sensitivity and body mass as predictors of fear during exercise. *Cognitive Behaviour Therapy, 39*, 28–36.

Chapter 4

1. Carver, C. S., & Scheier, M. F. (2008). Feedback processes in the simultaneous regulation of action and affect. In J. Y. Shah, & W. L. Gardner (Eds.), *Handbook of Motivational Science* (pp. 308–324). New York: Guilford.

2. Aarts, J., Dijksterhuis, A., & Dik, G. (2008). Goal contagion; inferring goals from others' actions–and what it leads to. In J. Y. Shah, & W. L. Gardner (Eds.), *Handbook of Motivational Science* (pp. 265–280). New York: Guilford.

3. King, A. C., Toobert, D., Ahn, D., Resnicow, K., Coday, M., Riebe, D., et al. (2006). Perceived environments as physical activity correlates and moderators of intervention in five studies. *American Journal of Health Promotion, 21*, 24–35.

4a. Carver, C. S., & Scheier, M. F. (2008). Feedback processes in the simultaneous regulation of action and affect. In J. Y. Shah, & W. L. Gardner (Eds.), *Handbook of Motivational Science* (pp. 308–324). New York: Guilford.

4b. Simon, H. A. (1967). Motivational and emotional controls of cognition. *Psychological Review, 74,* 29–39.

5. Orell, S., Hodgkins, S., & Sheeran, P. (1997). Implementation intentions and the theory of planned behavior. *Personality and Social Psychology Bulletin, 23,* 945–954.

6. Thaler, R. H., & Sustein, C. R. (2008). *Nudge: Improving decisions about health, wealth, and happiness.* New York: Penguin Books.

7. Example discussed by Thaler & Sustein (2008), with product information at http://www.urinalfly.com/

8. Muraven, M., & Baumeister, R. F. (2000). Self-regulation and depletion of limited resources: Does self-control resemble a muscle? *Psychological Bulletin, 126,* 147–259.

9. Thomas, D. L., & Diener, E. (1990). Memory accuracy in the recall of emotions. *Journal of Personality and Social Psychology, 59,* 291–297.

10. Kahneman, D., Fredrickson, B. L., Schreiber, C. A., & Redelmeier, D. A. (1993). When more pain is preferred to less: Adding a better end. *Psychological Science, 4,* 401–405.

11. Kwan, B. M., & Bryan, A. (2010). In-task and post-task affective response to exercise: Translating exercise intentions into behaviour. *British Journal of Health Psychology, 15,* 115–131.

12. Skinner, B. F. (1981). How to discover what you have to say—A talk to students. *The Behavior Analyst, 4,* 1–7.

13a. Annesi, J. J. (2004). Relationship of social cognitive theory factors to exercise maintenance in adults. *Perceptual and Motor Skills, 99,* 142–114.

13b. Moore, S. M., Dolansky, M. A., Ruland, C. M., Pashkow, F. J., & Blackburn, G. G. (2003). Predictors of women's exercise maintenance after cardiac rehabilitation. *Journal of Cardiopulmonary Rehabilitation, 23,* 40–49.

14a. Cialdini, R. B. (1984). *Influence: The psychology of persuasion* (Rev. ed.). New York: William Morrow and Co., Inc.

14b. Otto, M.W., Reilly-Harrington, N. A., Kogan, J. N., & Winett, C. A. (2003). Treatment contracting in cognitive-behavior therapy. *Cognitive and Behavioral Practice, 10,* 199–203.

Chapter 5

1. Loftus, E. F., & Palmer, J. C. (1974). Reconstruction of automobile destruction: An example of the interaction between language and memory. *Journal of Verbal Learning and Behavior, 13,* 585–589.

2. Peckham, A. D., McHugh, R. K., & Otto, M. W. (2010). A meta-analysis of the magnitude of biased attention in depression. *Depression and Anxiety. 27,* 1135–1142.

3a. Frewen, P. A., Dozois, D. J., Joanisse, M. F., & Neufeld, R. W. (2008). Selective attention to threat versus reward: Meta-analysis and neural-network modeling of the dot-probe task. *Clinical Psychology Review, 28*, 307–337.

3b. Clark, D. A., Beck, A. T., & Alford, B. A. (1999). *Scientific foundations of cognitive theory and therapy of depression.* Philadelphia: John Wiley & Sons.

4a. Fava, M., Bless, E., Otto, M. W., Pava, J. A., & Rosenbaum, J. F. (1994). Dysfunctional attitudes in major depression: Changes with pharmacotherapy. *Journal of Nervous and Mental Disease, 182*, 45–49.

4b. Clark, D. A., Beck, A. T., & Alford, B. A. (1999). *Scientific foundations of cognitive theory and therapy of depression.* Philadelphia: John Wiley & Sons.

5. Otto, M. W., Fava, M., Penava, S. A., Bless, E., Muller, R. T., & Rosenbaum, J. F. (1997). Life event and cognitive predictors of perceived stress before and after treatment for major depression. *Cognitive Therapy and Research, 21*, 409–420.

6. Source: OAG Aviation & PlaneCrashInfo.com accident database, 1985–2009.

7. Clark, D. A., & Beck, A. T. (2010). *Cognitive therapy of anxiety disorders: Science and practice.* New York: Guilford Press.

7a. Clark D. A., Beck, A. T., & Alford, B. A. (1999). *Scientific foundations of cognitive theory and therapy of depression.* Philadelphia: John Wiley & Sons.
Self-help books that emphasize a cognitive therapy approach include books such as:

7b. Burns, D. D. (1980). *Feeling good: The new mood therapy* (Rev. & updated ed.). New York: Avon Books.

7c. Ellis, A., & Harper, R. A. (1997). *A guide to rational living.* Chatsworth, CA: Wilshire Book Company.

7d. Leahy, R. L. (2005). *The worry cure: Seven steps to stop worry from stopping you.* New York: Three Rivers Press.

8. Story is adapted from Otto, M. W. (2000). Stories and metaphors in cognitive-behavior therapy. *Cognitive and Behavioral Practice, 7*, 166–172.

9. Tice, D. M., & Baumeister, R. F. (1997). Longitudinal study of procrastination, performance, stress, and health: The costs and benefits of dawdling. *Psychological Science, 8*, 454–458.

10. Weiner, B. (1985). An attributional theory of achievement motivation and emotion. *Psychological Review, 92*, 548–573.

11. Smith, P. J., Blumenthal, J. A., Hoffman, B. M., Cooper, H., Strauman, T. A., Welsh-Bohmer K., et al. (2010). Aerobic exercise and neurocognitive performance: A meta-analytic review of randomized controlled trials. *Psychosomatic Medicine, 72*, 239–252.

Chapter 6

1. Edwards, B. J., Edwards, W., Waterhouse, J., Atkinson, G., & Reilly, T. (2005). Can cycling performance in an early morning, laboratory-based cycle time-trial

be improved by morning exercise the day before? *International Journal of Sports Medicine, 26,* 651–656.

2. Atkinson, G., & Reilly, T. (1996). Circadian variation in sports performance. *Sports Medicine, 21,* 292–312.

3. This concept has been emphasized in treatments for insomnia, where good planning can be compromised by a wishful sleepy mind: see Perlis, M. L., Jungquist, C., Smith, M. T., & Posner, D. (2005). *Cognitive-behavioral treatment of insomnia: A step by step guide.* New York: Springer.

4. Atkinson, G., & Reilly, T. (1996). Circadian variation in sports performance. *Sports Medicine, 21,* 292–312.

5. Smith, P. J., Blumenthal, J. A., Hoffman, B. M., Cooper, H., Strauman, T. A., Welsh-Bohmer, K., et al. (2010). Aerobic exercise and neurocognitive performance: A meta-analytic review of randomized controlled trials. *Psychosomatic Medicine, 72,* 239–252.

6. Middleton, L. E., Barnes, D. E., Lui, L. Y., & Yaffe, K. (2010). Physical activity over the life course and its association with cognitive performance and impairment in old age. *Journal of American Geriatric Society, 58,* 1322–1326.

7a. Sofi, F., Capalbo, A., Marcucci, R., Gori, A. M., Fedi, S., Macchi, C., et al. (2007). Leisure time but not occupational physical activity significantly affects cardiovascular risk factors in an adult population. *European Journal of Clinical Investigation, 37,* 947–953.

7b. Oppert, J. M., Thomas, F., Charles, M. A., Benetos, A., Basdevant, A., & Simon, C. (2006). Leisure-time and occupational physical activity in relation to cardiovascular risk factors and eating habits in French adults. *Public Health Nutrition, 9,* 746–754.

7c. Pols, M. A., Peeters, P. H. M., Twisk, J. W. R., Kemper, H. C. G., & Grobbee, D. E. (1997). Physical activity and cardiovascular disease risk profile in women. *American Journal of Epidemiology, 146,* 322–328.

8. Smith, P. J., Blumenthal, J. A., Hoffman, B. M., Cooper, H., Strauman, T. A., Welsh-Bohmer, K., et al. (2010). Aerobic exercise and neurocognitive performance: A meta-analytic review of randomized controlled trials. *Psychosomatic Medicine, 72,* 239–252.

9. We don't know the source of this saying, but it seems to be ubiquitous, in some form, to web pages everywhere.

10. Kwan, B. M., Bryan, A. (2010). In-task and post-task affective response to exercise: Translating exercise intentions into behaviour. *British Journal of Health Psychology, 15*(1), 115–131.

Chapter 7

1. American College of Sports Medicine. (2005). *ACSM's guidelines for exercise testing and prescription* (6th ed.). Philadelphia: Lippincott Williams, & Wilkins.

2. Shephard, R. J., Cox, M. H., & Simper, K. (1981). An analysis of "Par-Q" responses in an office population. *Canadian Journal of Public Health, 72,* 37–40.

3. http://www.cdc.gov/physicalactivity/everyone/measuring/index.html

4. Physical Activity Guidelines Advisory Committee. (2008). *Physical activity guidelines advisory committee report, 2008.* Washington, DC: U.S. Department of Health and Human Services.

5. Stathopoulou, G., Powers, M. B., Berry, A. C., Smits, J. A. J., & Otto, M. W. (2006). Exercise interventions for mental health: A quantitative and qualitative review. *Clinical Psychology: Science & Practice, 13,* 179–193.

6. Physical Activity Guidelines Advisory Committee. (2008). *Physical Activity Guidelines Advisory Committee report, 2008.* Washington, DC: U.S. Department of Health and Human Services.

7. Physical Activity Guidelines Advisory Committee. (2008). *Physical Activity Guidelines Advisory Committee report, 2008.* Washington, DC: U.S. Department of Health and Human Services.

8. American College of Sports Medicine. (2005). *ACSM's guidelines for exercise testing and prescription* (6th ed.). Philadelphia: Lippincott Williams, & Wilkins.

9a. Shilts, M. K., Horowitz, M., & Townsend, M. S. (2004). Goal setting as a strategy for dietary and physical activity behavior change: A review of the literature. *American Journal of Health Promotion, 19,* 81–93.

9. Shilts, M. K., Horowitz, M., Townsend, M. S. (2009). Guided goal setting: Effectiveness in a dietary and physical activity intervention with low-income adolescents. *International Journal of Adolescent Medical Health, 21,* 111–122.

10. McAuley, E., & Blissmer, B. (2000). Self-efficacy determinants and consequences of physical activity. *Exercise and Sport Science Review, 28,* 85–88.

11. Cialdini, R. B. (1984). *Influence: The psychology of persuasion* (Rev. ed.). New York: William Morrow and Co., Inc.

12a. Izawa, K. P., Watanabe, S., Omiya, K., Hirano, Y., Oka, K., Osada, N., & Iijima, S. (2005). Effect of the self-monitoring approach on exercise maintenance during cardiac rehabilitation: A randomized, controlled trial. *American Journal of Physical Medicine & Rehabilitation, 84,* 313–321.

12b. Carels, R. A., Darby, L. A., Rydin, S., Douglass, O. M., Cacciapaglia, H. M., & O'Brien, W. H. (2005). The relationship between self-monitoring, outcome expectancies, difficulties with eating and exercise, and physical activity and weight loss treatment outcomes. *Annals of Behavioral Medicine, 30,* 182–190.

Chapter 8

1. Strack, F., Martin, L., & Stepper, S. (1988). Inhibiting and facilitating conditions of the human smile: A non-obtrusive test of the facial feedback hypothesis. *Journal of Personality and Social Psychology, 54,* 768–777.

2. Davis, J. I., Senghas, A., Brandt, F., & Ochsner, K. N. (2010). The effects of BOTOX injections on emotional experience. *Emotion, 10*, 433–440.

3a. Kabat-Zinn, J. (1994). *Wherever you go, there you are: Mindfulness meditation in everyday life*. New York: Hyperion.

3b. Germer, C. K., Siegel, R. D., & Fulton, P. R (Eds.). (2005). *Mindfulness and Psychotherapy*. Guilford Press: New York.

4a. Stathopoulou, G., Powers, M. B., Berry, A. C., Smits, J. A. J., & Otto, M. W. (2006). Exercise interventions for mental health: A quantitative and qualitative review. *Clinical Psychology: Science and Practice, 13*, 179–193.

4b. Kodama, S., Saito, K., Tanaka, S., Maki, M., Yachi, Y., Asumi, M., et al. (2009). Cardiorespiratory fitness as a quantitative predictor of all-cause mortality and cardiovascular events in healthy men and women: A meta-analysis. *Journal of the American Medical Association, 301*, 2024–2035.

4c. Berlin, J. A., & Colditz, G. A. (1990). A meta-analysis of physical activity in the prevention of coronary heart disease. *American Journal of Epidemiology, 134*, 232–234.

5a. Smits, J. A. J., Powers, M. B., Utschig, A. C., & Otto, M. W. (2007). Translating empirically-supported strategies into accessible interventions: The potential utility of exercise for the treatment of panic disorder. *Cognitive and Behavioral Practice, 14*, 364–374.

5b. Broocks, A., Bandelow, B., Pekrun, G., George, A., Meyer, T., Bartman, U., et al. (1998). Comparison of aerobic exercise, clomipramine, and placebo in the treatment of panic disorder. *American Journal of Psychiatry, 155*, 603–609.

6. Otto, M. W., & Smits, J. A. J. (2009). *Exercise for mood and anxiety disorders: Workbook* (p. 71). New York: Oxford University Press.

7. From "Nothing Gold Can Stay" by Robert Frost.

7a. Levin, D. (1982.). The runner's high: Fact or fiction? *The Journal of the American Medical Association, 248*(1), 24.

7b. Partin, C. (1983). Runner's high. *The Journal of the American Medical Association, 249*(1), 21.

8a. Carr, D. B., Bullen, B. A., Skrinar, G. S., Arnold, M. A., Rosenblatt, M., Beitins, I. Z., et al. (1981). Physical conditioning facilitates the exercise-induced secretion of β-endorphin and β-lipotropin in women. *New England Journal of Medicine, 305*, 560–563.

8b. Schwarz, L., & Kindermann, W. (1992). Changes in beta-endorphin levels in response to aerobic and anaerobic exercise. *Sports Medicine, 13*, 25–36.

Chapter 9

1. Peckham, A. D., McHugh, R. K., & Otto, M. W. (2010). A meta-analysis of the magnitude of biased attention in depression. *Depression and Anxiety, 27*, 1135–1142.

2. Smits, J. A. J., & Otto, M. W. (2009). *Exercise for mood and anxiety disorders: Therapist guide* (pp. 62–64). New York: Oxford University Press. (reprinted with permission).

3. Michie, S., Abraham, C., Whittington, C., McAteer, J., & Gupta, S. (2009). Effective techniques in healthy eating and physical activity interventions: A meta-regression. *Health Psychology, 28,* 690–701.

4. Rush, A. J., Trivedi, M. H., Ibrahim, H. M., Carmody, T. J., Arnow, B., Klein, D. N., et al. (2003). The 16-item Quick Inventory of Depressive Symptomatology (QIDS) clinician rating (QIDS-C) and self-report (QIDS-SR): A psychometric evaluation in patients with chronic major depression. *Biological Psychiatry, 54,* 573–583.

5a. Church, T. S., Martin, C. K., Thompson, A. M., Earnest, C. P., Mikus, C. R., & Blair, S. N. (2009). Changes in weight, waist circumference and compensatory responses with different doses of exercise among sedentary, overweight postmenopausal women. *PLoS One, 4*(2), e4515.

5b. Donnelly, J. E., & Smith, B. K. (2005). Is exercise effective for weight loss with ad libitum diet? Energy balance, compensation, and gender differences. *Exercise and Sport Sciences Reviews, 33,* 169–174.

6. Chernev, A. (in press). The dieter's paradox, *Journal of Consumer Psychology.* See also Chandon, P., & Wansink, B. (2007). The biasing health halos of fast-food restaurant health claims: Lower calorie estimates and higher side-dish consumption intentions. *Journal of Consumer Research, 34,* 301–314.

7. Patel, A. V., Bernstein, L., Deka, A., Feigelson, H. S., Campbell, P. T., Gapstur, S. M., et al. (2010). Leisure time spent sitting in relation to total mortality in a prospective cohort of US adults. *American Journal of Epidemiology, 172,* 419–429.

8. Warren, T. Y., Barry, V., Hooker, S.P., Sui, X., Church, T. S., Blair, S. N. (2010). Sedentary behaviors increase risk of cardiovascular disease mortality in men. *Medicine and Science in Sports & Exercise, 42,* 879–885.

9. Healy, G. N., Dunstan, D. W., Salmon, J., Cerin, E., Shaw, J. E., Zimmet, P. Z., & Owen, N. (2008). Breaks in sedentary time: Beneficial associations with metabolic risk. *Diabetes Care, 31,* 661–666.

10. A note of thanks to Roger Moore, Ph.D. who discussed this idea years ago.

11a. Levine, J. A., Eberhardt, N. L., & Jensen, M. D. (1999). Role of nonexercise activity thermogenesis in resistance to fat gain in humans. *Science, 283*(5399), 212–214.

11b. Levine, J. A., Schleusner, S. J., & Jensen, M. D. Energy expenditure of nonexercise activity. *American Journal of Clinical Nutrition, 72,* 1451–1454.

12. Katz, M. (2008, September 16). I put in 5 miles at the office. *New York Times,* G8.

13. Levine J. A., & Miller, J. M. (2007). The energy expenditure of using a "walk-and-work" desk for office workers with obesity. *British Journal of Sports Medicine, 41,* 558–561.

Chapter 10

1. Williams, D. M., Dunsiger, S., Ciccolo, J. T., Lewis, B. A., Albrecht, A. E., & Marcus, B. H. (2008). Acute affective response to a moderate-intensity

exercise stimulus predicts physical activity participation 6 and 12 months later. *Psychology of Sport and Exercise, 9,* 231–245.

2. Stanley, D.M., & Cumming, J. (2010). Are we having fun yet? Testing the effects of imagery use on the affective and enjoyment responses to acute moderate exercise. *Psychology of Sport and Exercise, 11,* 582–590.

3. Nakamura, P. M., Pereira, G., Papini, C. B., Nakamura, F. Y., & Kokubun, E. (2010). Effects of preferred and nonpreferred music on continuous cycling exercise performance. *Perceptual and Motor Skills, 110,* 257–264.

4. Gibala, M. J., & McGee, S. L. (2008). Metabolic adaptations to short-term high-intensity interval training: A little pain for a lot of gain? *Exercise and Sports Sciences Review, 36,* 58–63.

5. Babraj, J. A., Vollaard, N. B., Keast, C., Guppy, F. M., Cottrell, G., & Timmons, J. A. (2009). Extremely short duration high intensity interval training substantially improves insulin action in young healthy males. *BMC Endocrine Disorder, 9,* 3.

6. Talanian, J. L., Galloway, S. D., Heigenhauser, G. J., Bonen, A., & Spriet, L. L. (2007). Two weeks of high-intensity aerobic interval training increases the capacity for fat oxidation during exercise in women. *Journal of Applied Physiology, 102,* 1439–1447.

7. Kübler-Ross, E. (1973). *On death and dying,* Oxford, UK: Routledge.

8a. Dutton, D., & Aron, A. P. (1974). Some evidence for heightened sexual attraction under conditions of high anxiety. *Journal of Personality and Social Psychology, 23,* 510–517.

8b. Foster, C. A., Witcher, B. S., Campbell, W. K., & Green, J. D. (1998). Arousal and attraction: Evidence for automatic and controlled processes. *Journal of Personality and Social Psychology, 74,* 86–101.

9. Weissman, M. M., Wolk, S., Goldstein, R. B., Moreau, D., Adams, P., Greenwald, S., et al. (1999). Depressed adolescents grown up. *Journal of the American Medical Association, 281,* 1707–1713.

10a. Richardson, L. P., Davis, R., Poulton, R., McCauley, E., Moffitt, T. E., Caspi, A., & Connell, F. (2003). A longitudinal evaluation of adolescent depression and adult obesity. *Archives of Pediatric and Adolescent Medicine, 157,* 739–745.

10b. Pine, D. S., Cohen, P., Brook, J., & Coplan, J. D. (1997). Psychiatric symptoms in adolescence as predictors of obesity in early adulthood: A longitudinal study. *American Journal of Public Health, 87,* 1303–1310.

11. Jacka, F. N., Pasco, J. A., Mykletun, A., Williams, L. J., Hodge, A. M., O'Reilly, S. L., et al. (2010). Association of Western and Traditional diets with depression and anxiety in women. *American Journal of Psychiatry, 167,* 1–7.

12. Kimm, S. Y., Glynn, N. W., Kriska, A. M., Barton, B. A., Kronsberg, S. S., Daniels, S. R., et al. (2002). Decline in physical activity in black girls and white girls during adolescence. *New England Journal of Medicine, 347,* 709–715.

13a. Update: Prevalence of overweight among children, adolescents, and adults—United States, 1988-1994. (1997). *MMWR: Morbidity and Mortality Weekly Report, 46,* 198–202.

13b. Dietz, W. H., & Gortmaker S. L. (2001). Preventing obesity in children and adolescents. *Annual Review of Public Health, 22,* 337–353.

14. Singh, G. K., Kogan, M. D., van Dyck, P. C. (2010). Changes in state-specific childhood obesity and overweight prevalence in the United States from 2003 to 2007. *Archives of Pediatric Adolescent Medicine, 164,* 598–607.

15a. Freedman, D. S., Dietz, W. H., Srinivasan, S. R., & Berenson, G. S. (1999). The relation of overweight to cardiovascular risk factors among children and adolescents: The Bogalusa Heart Study. *Pediatrics, 103*(6 Pt 1), 1175–1182.

15b. Sinha, R., Fisch, G., Teague, B., Tamborlane, W. V., Banyas, B., Allen, K., et al. (2002). Prevalence of impaired glucose tolerance among children and adolescents with marked obesity. *New England Journal of Medicine, 346,* 802–810.

16. Griffiths, L. J., Dowda, M., Dezateux, C., & Pate, R. (2010). Associations between sport and screen-entertainment with mental health problems in 5-year-old children. *International Journal of Behavioral Nutrition and Physical Activity, 7,* 30–41.

17. Stevenson, B. (2010). Beyond the classroom: Using Title IX to measure the return to high school sports. *Review of Economics and Statistics,* May, 284–301.

18. Hill, L., Williams, J. H., Aucott, L., Milne, J., Thomson, J., Greig, J., et al. (2010). Exercising attention within the classroom. *Development Medicine and Child Neurology, 52,* 929–934.[Epub ahead of print]

19. Smith, P. J., Blumenthal, J. A., Hoffman, B. M., Cooper, H., Strauman, T. A., Welsh-Bohmer, K., et al. (2010). Aerobic exercise and neurocognitive performance: A meta-analytic review of randomized controlled trials. *Psychosomatic Medicine, 72,* 239–252.

20. Allender, S., Cowburn, G., & Foster, C. (2006). Understanding participation in sport and physical activity among children and adults: A review of qualitative studies. *Health Education Research: Theory & Practice, 21,* 826–835.

21. Good advice from the Women's Sport Foundation. Retrieved from http://www.womenssportsfoundation.org

22. Boiche, J. C. S., Sarrazin, P. G., Grouzet, F. M. E., Pelletier, L. G., & Chanal, J. P. (2008). Students' motivational profiles and achievement outcomes in physical education: A self-determination perspective. *Journal of Educational Psychology, 100,* 688–701.

23a. Bamber, D. J., Cockeril, I. M., Rodgers, S., & Carroll, D. (2003). Diagnostic criteria for exercise dependence in women. *British Journal of Sports Medicine, 37,* 393–400.

23b. Torstveit, M. K., & Sundgot-Borgen, J. (2005). The female athlete triad exists in both elite athletes and controls. *Medicine and Science in Sports & Exercise, 37,* 1449–1459.

23c. West, R. V. (1998). The female athlete. The triad of disordered eating, amenorrhoea and osteoporosis. *Sports Medicine, 26,* 63–71.

24a. Stice, E., Rohde, P., Gau, J., & Shaw, H. An effectiveness trial of a dissonance-based eating disorder prevention program for high-risk adolescent girls. *Journal of Consulting and Clinical Psychology, 77,* 825–834.

24b. Stice, E., Shaw, H., Becker, C. B., & Rohde, P. (2008). Dissonance-based interventions for the prevention of eating disorders: Using persuasion principles to promote health. *Prevention Science, 9,* 114–128.

24c. Also see eatingforlifealliance.org.

Chapter 11

1. Martin, C. K., Church, T. S., Thompson, A. M., Earnest, C. P., & Blair, S. N. (2009). Exercise dose and quality of life: A randomized controlled trial. *Archives of Internal Medicine, 169,* 269–278.

2. Kodama, S., Saito, K., Tanaka, S., Maki, M., Yachi, Y., Asumi, M., et al. (2009). Cardiorespiratory fitness as a quantitative predictor of all-cause mortality and cardiovascular events in healthy men and women: A meta-analysis. *Journal of the American Medical Association, 301,* 2024–2035.

3a. Lee, C. D., Blair, S. N., & Jackson, A. S. (1999). Cardiorespiratory fitness, body composition, and all-cause and cardiovascular disease mortality in men. *American Journal of Clinical Nutrition, 69,* 373–380.

3b. Borodulin, K., Laatikainen, T., Lahti-Koski, M., Lakka, T. A., Laukkanen, R., Sarna, S., & Jousilahti, P. (2005). Associations between estimated aerobic fitness and cardiovascular risk factors in adults with different levels of abdominal obesity. *European Journal of Cardiovascular Prevention and Rehabilitation, 12,* 126–131.

4. Singh, G. K., Kogan, M. D., & van Dyck, P. C. (2010). Changes in state-specific childhood obesity and overweight prevalence in the United States from 2003 to 2007. *Archives of Pediatric and Adolescent Medicine, 164,* 598–607.

5. Christakis, N. A., & Fowler, J. H. (2007). The spread of obesity in a large social network over 32 years. *New England Journal of Medicine, 357,* 370–379.

6a. Jansen, A., Vanreyten, A., van Balveren, T., Roefs, A., & Nederkoorn, C. (2008). Negative affect and cue-induced overeating in non-eating disordered obesity. *Appetite, 51,* 556–562.

6b. Dingemans, A. E., Martijn, C., Jansen, A. T., van Furth, E. F. (2009). The effect of suppressing negative emotions on eating behavior in binge eating disorder. *Appetite, 52,* 51–57.

7. Jacka, F. N., Pasco, J. A., Mykletun, A., Williams, L. J., Hodge, A. M., O'Reilly, S. L., et al. (2010). Association of Western and Traditional diets with depression and anxiety in women. *American Journal of Psychiatry, 167,* 1–7.

8a. Tice, D. M., Batslavsky, E., & Baumeiser, R. F. (2001). Emotional distress regulation takes precedence over impulse control. If you feel bad, do it! *Journal of Personality and Social Psychology, 8*, 53–67.

8b. Jansen, A., Vanreyten, A., van Balveren, T., Roefs, A., & Nederkoorn, C. (2008). Negative affect and cue-induced overeating in non-eating disordered obesity. *Appetite, 51*, 556–562.

8c. Dingemans, A. E., Martijn, C., Jansen, A. T., & van Furth, E. F. (2009). The effect of suppressing negative emotions on eating behavior in binge eating disorder. *Appetite, 52*, 51–57.

9. Tice, D. M., Batslavsky, E., & Baumeiser, R. F. (2001). Emotional distress regulation takes precedence over impulse control. If you feel bad, do it! *Journal of Personality and Social Psychology, 8*, 53–67.

10a. Sánchez-Villegas, A., Delgado-Rodríguez, M., Alonso, A., Schlatter, J., Lahortiga, F., Serra Majem, L., Martínez-González, M. A. (2009). Association of the Mediterranean dietary pattern with the incidence of depression: the Seguimiento Universidad de Navarra/University of Navarra follow-up (SUN) cohort. *Archives of General Psychiatry, 66*, 1090–1098.

10b. Akbarly, T. N., Brunner, E. J., Ferrie, J. E., Marmot, M. G., Kivimaki, M., & Singh-Manoux, A. (2009). Dietary pattern and depressive symptoms in middle age. *British Journal of Psychiatry, 195*, 408–413.

11a. Sofi, F., Abbate, R., Gensini, G. F., & Casini, A. (2010). Accruing evidence about benefits of adherence to the Mediterranean diet on health: An updated systematic review and meta analysis. *American journal of Clinical Nutrition, 92*, 1189–1196.

11b. Sofi, F., Cesari, F., Abbate, R., Gensini, G. F., & Casini, A. (2008). Adherence to Mediterranean diet and health status: Meta-analysis. *British Medical Journal, 337*, a1344. doi:10.1136/bmj.a1344

12a. Booth, S. L., Sallis, J. F., Ritenbaugh, C., Hill, J. O., Birch, L. L., Frank, L. D., et al. (2001). Environmental and societal factors affect food choice and physical activity: Rationale, influences, and leverage points. *Nutrition Review, 3*, 21–39.

12b. Wansink, B. (2004). Environmental factors that increase the food intake and consumption volume of unknowing consumers. *Annual Review of Nutrition, 24*, 455–479.

13. Painter J. E., Wansink B., & Hieggelke, J. B. (2002). How visibility and convenience influence candy consumption. *Appetite, 38*, 237–238.

14. Wansink, B., & Cheney, M. M. (2005). Super bowls: Serving bowl size and food consumption. *Journal of the American Medical Association, 293*, 1727–1728.

15. Wansink, B. (2004). Environmental factors that increase the food intake and consumption volume of unknowing consumers. *Annual Review of Nutrition, 24*, 455–479.

16. Putnam, R. D. (2000). *Bowling alone: The collapse and revival of American community*. New York: Simon & Schuster.

17a. Taylor, C. T., Bomyea, J., & Amir, N. (2010). Attentional bias away from positive social information mediates the link between social anxiety and anxiety vulnerability to a social stressor. *Journal of Anxiety Disorders, 24,* 403–408.

17b. Amir, N., Beard, C., Burns, M., & Bomyea, J. (2009). Attention modification program in individuals with generalized anxiety disorder. *Journal of Abnormal Psychology, 118,* 28–33.

18a. Bureau of Labor Statistics (2010). American Time Use Survey Summary (2009 Results), http://www.bls.gov/news.release/atus.nr0.htm

18b. Raynor, D. A., Phelan, S., Hill, J. O., & Wing, R. R. (2006). Television viewing and longterm weight maintenance: Results from the National Weight Control Registry. *Obesity, 14,* 1816–1824.

19. Fowler, J. H., Christakis, N. A. (2008). Dynamic spread of happiness in a large social network: Longitudinal analysis over 20 years in the Framingham Heart Study. *British Medical Journal, 337,* a2338. doi:10.1136/bmj.a2338

20. Rosenquist, J. N., Fowler, J. H., Christakis, N. A. (2011). Social network determinants of depression. *Molecular Psychiatry, 16,* 273–281.

INDEX

ABOUT THE AUTHORS

Michael W. Otto, Ph.D. is Professor of Psychology at Boston University. He is a behavior-change expert who has done extensive research on strategies to improve treatments for anxiety, mood, and substance use disorders.

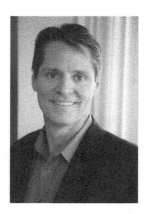

Photo credit: Allison Evans

Jasper A. J. Smits, Ph.D. is Associate Professor of Psychology at Southern Methodist University. His research focuses on the development of interventions, including exercise, for anxiety disorders and smoking.

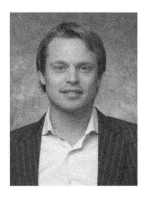

Photo credit: Hillsman Jackson